THE
HOW NOT TO DIE
COOKBOOK

THE HOW NO
COOKBOOK

MICHAEL GREGER, M.D., FACLM

WITH Gene Stone

RECIPES BY Robin Robertson

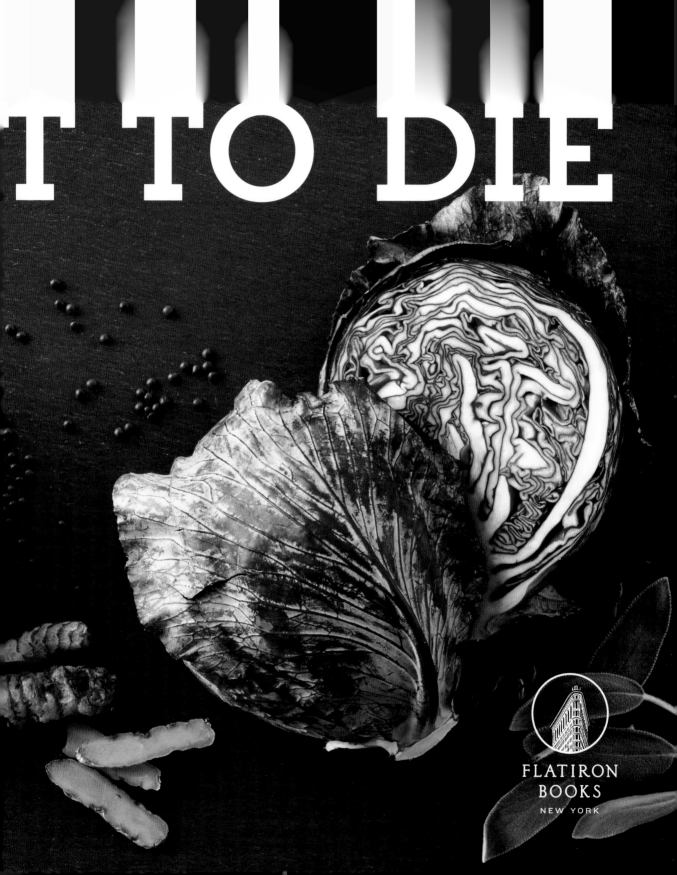

T TO DIE

FLATIRON
BOOKS
NEW YORK

The How Not to Die Cookbook. Copyright © 2017 by Michael Greger with Gene Stone. All rights reserved. Printed in China.
For information, address Flatiron Books, 175 Fifth Avenue, New York, NY 10010.

www.flatironbooks.com

Produced by Print Matters Productions, Inc.

Photography by Antonis Achilleos

Interior design by Alison Lew/Vertigo Design NYC

Cover design by Jason Gabbert

Cover photography: blueberries © Audrius Merfeldas / Shutterstock; cilantro licensed under CC by 4.0 from Vegetables Fridge Alphabet (http://foodfont.com/vegetables-fridge) by Kristen Baumlier; tomatillos/onions licensed under CC by 4.0 from Veggies Fall Farmers@Firehouse Alphabet (http://foodfont.com/veggies-fall) by Visitors to the Farmers@Firehouse Market; tomatoes and green beans licensed under CC by 4.0 from Summer Vegetable Gordon Square Market Alphabet (http://foodfont.com/summer-vegetable) by Visitors to the Gordon Square Market Alphabet

The Library of Congress Cataloging-in-Publication Data is available upon request.

ISBN 978-1-250-12776-1 (hardcover)
ISBN 978-1-250-12775-4 (e-book)

Our books may be purchased in bulk for promotional, educational, or business use. Please contact your local bookseller or the Macmillan Corporate and Premium Sales Department at 1-800-221-7945, extension 5442, or by e-mail at MacmillanSpecialMarkets@macmillan.com.

First Edition: December 2017

10 9 8 7 6 5 4 3 2 1

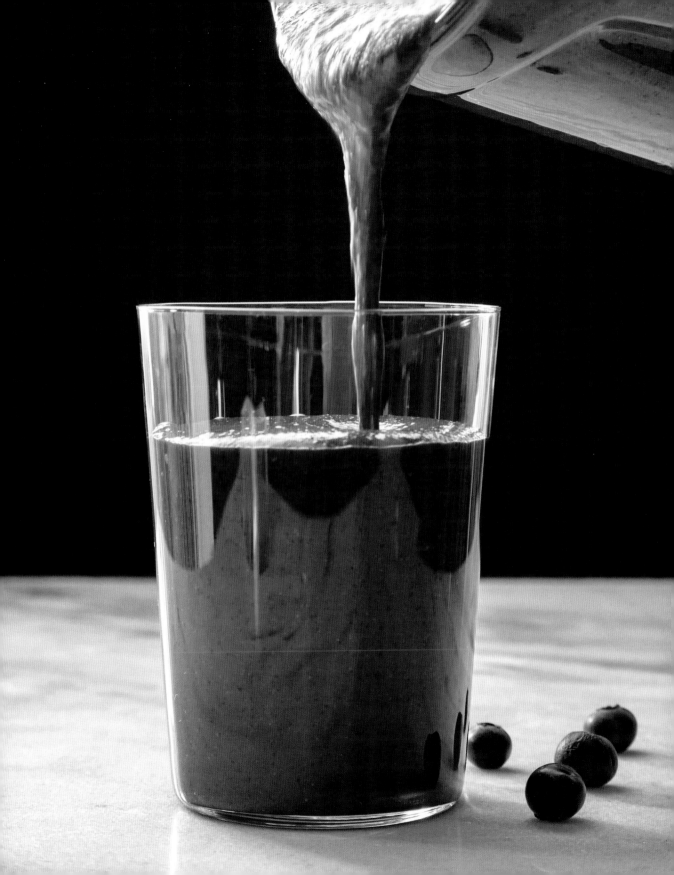

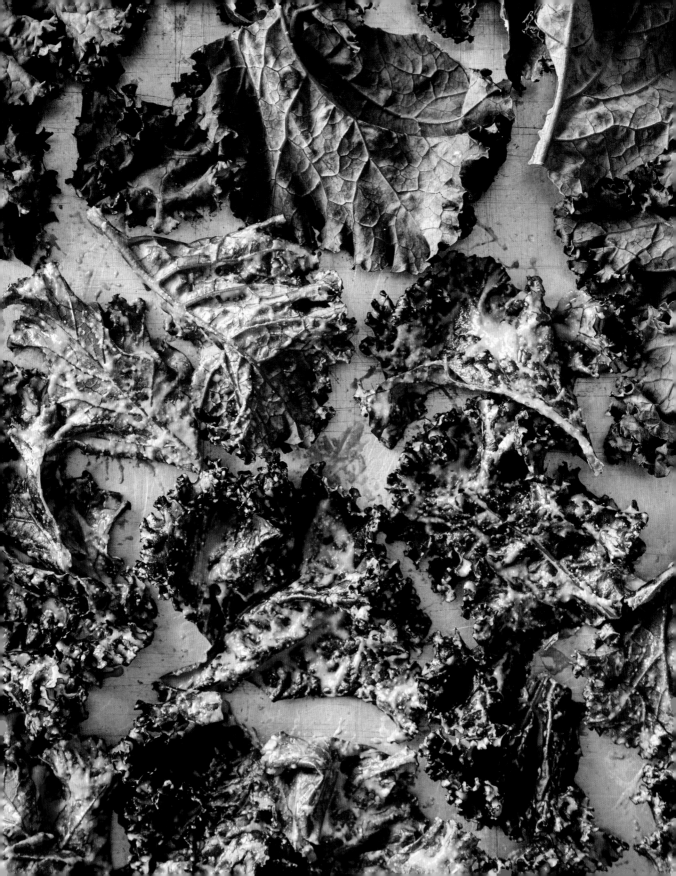

CONTENTS

Introduction viii

The Daily Dozen xx

ONE **SIMPLE PREPARATIONS** 1

TWO **BREAKFAST** 10

THREE **SNACKS, DIPS, AND SPREADS** 28

FOUR **SOUPS AND CHILIES** 46

FIVE **SALADS AND DRESSINGS** 68

SIX **BURGERS, WRAPS, AND MORE** 86

SEVEN **VERY VEGGIE MAINS** 102

EIGHT **BEAN CUISINE** 122

NINE **GREAT GRAINS** 140

TEN **SIDES** 162

ELEVEN **SWEETS** 184

TWELVE **SIPS** 204

Sample Menus for 14 Days 220

Kitchen Techniques 225

Shopping and Stocking the Pantry 227

References 230

Index 237

INTRODUCTION

I admit it.

I am a nutrition nerd. I love digging through the scientific literature for the fun of it, for the sheer fascination of how our body works, for all the puzzles to be solved. In high school, I used to skip class to hang out in the science library at the local university, spending countless hours trying to read the new issues of all the journals. I hardly understood any of it, but I just loved the whole concept of scientific inquiry: using experimental evidence to test our theories about the universe.

In college, I pursued a biophysics major. I was most interested in the mysteries of the universe inside each of us. As enthralling as all of science and mathematics was, I came to realize that our number one cause of death and disability wasn't the Higgs boson—it was our diet. My mother's deep involvement in the civil rights movement inspired me to dedicate my life to making the world a better place, and my grandmother's miraculous recovery from end-stage heart disease, due to a change in her diet, provided the direction: I would become a doctor and specialize in nutrition.

Even if it didn't help a soul, though, I could happily spend seven days a week lost in the dusty stacks of some medical library basement to satisfy my own curiosity. But what most motivates me every morning to jump out of bed (and onto my treadmill desk!) are all the lives I'm able to help change and save with the information I uncover. For years, my work had touched millions through NutritionFacts.org, but it wasn't until *How Not to Die* was published that the deluge started. My inbox, mailbox, and voice-mail box have been flooded with profound expressions of gratitude from readers telling me how the science I've shared has helped them and their families become healthier. They are such a gift.

Even better is to experience that appreciation for my work face-to-face and heart-to-heart. As I've traveled around the world to share the book, I've been witness to countless stories of transformation. So many people line up to talk with me after my lectures that sometimes it can be several hours before I can dash back to the airport.

The stories often shared with me are not the ones most doctors hear, tales of pain and sickness. These are stories of regained health and happy endings. What could be more satisfying—for both of us?

Let me share one of these stories with you.

I met Chris, a middle-aged man, after a presentation I gave in Boston at Harvard's Dana-Farber Cancer Institute, where he was employed. Chris had come to my talk because although his type 2 diabetes diagnosis was about ten years old, he wasn't willing to settle for a lifetime of medication and monitoring as his doctor contended was to be his fate.

His physician had told him his diabetes was probably just the result of bad genes and Chris would need to take pills, adding he should "watch his sugar" (whatever that means). Chris knew diabetes was linked to such complications as blindness and amputations, and his doctor didn't seem very optimistic about the prognosis, nor did he offer any other recommendations.

Ten years earlier, Chris left his doctor's office feeling hopeless and helpless. He felt that he had just been given a death sentence. But he never stopped trying to seek out other answers, which brought him to my lecture.

After Chris recounted his experience, I told him that despite what his doctor might think, we actually have tremendous power over our health destiny. The vast majority of premature death and disability is preventable with a plant-based diet and other healthy lifestyle changes, and type 2 diabetes is a perfect example of a correctable disease.

Chris then handed me a copy of *How Not to Die* to autograph. As I always do when signing books, I included my personal e-mail address and cell phone number, and encouraged him to contact me if there was anything I could do to help him or his family.

About ten months later, Chris sent me this e-mail:

> *Dear Doc,*
> *You won't believe this. My diabetes is GONE. I beat it, doc!* How Not to Die *really did save my life! Guess what else? My wife has had problems with her weight since she was a teenager. We went on a plant-based diet together, and she has, for the first time in years, gotten to a normal weight! We are both so happy, we feel like teenagers again. (Did I tell you we were high school sweethearts? That was a very long time ago, but it doesn't feel so long ago anymore!)*

> *Also I want to mention that this diet is saving us some serious cash! I used to spend over $70 per month on my diabetes medications, my sugar meter, and test strip supplies. Now we are putting that money saved on medicine into . . . guess what . . . a Happiness Savings Account!*

> *We have both always wanted a dog, and when I finally beat diabetes, my wife said, "Your getting your health back is the best day of my life. We should celebrate it." And I told her I wanted to go to the shelter and get a dog. When the staff at the shelter asked what kind of dog we wanted, I said, "A nice dog who you don't think anyone else will want. The dog who everyone else gave up on. Second-chance dog, that's MY dog, please."*

> *The shelter folks talked for a minute, and then they brought out a big black dog with her head down and her tail tucked between her legs. We took one look at each other. Found out her name was Joy. Strange name for a sad dog, right? Well, we bonded fast, and now Joy, my wife, and I walk together every morning. We call it our JoyWalk! Joy is now living up to her name, and I think she saved me as much as I saved her.*

> *Most days I find all these new healthy choices easy, but when I get sidetracked, I just look at my Joy and remember how things were, and I remind myself that we are never going back there.*

> *Thank you for talking to me and for caring about me and my family. You will never know how much it means to me. I hope you can tell everyone what you told me about genes NOT being our destiny. There is hope and (at least in my house) there is Joy! Thanks, Dr. Greger!*

You're welcome, Chris!

Not everyone is so magnanimous, though. Others are angry. Why didn't their doctor tell them about how lifesaving our dietary choices can be? When I present decades-old studies showing how easily some of our leading killers can be reversed, the audience is left thinking, "Wait a second. Does that mean my brother didn't have to die?!" Or their sister or mother or best friend. Dr. Dean Ornish was publishing studies back in the 1990s proving heart disease could be reversed.[1] The diabetes reversal study I presented at the event Chris attended was published in 1979. It showed that people who had been living with type 2 diabetes for as long as twenty years, injecting up to 32 units of insulin a day, could get off all their insulin in as few as thirteen days.[2]

Let that sink in for a moment: People with diabetes for twenty years can go off all insulin in less than two weeks. They endured diabetes for twenty years because no one had told them about a plant-based diet. For decades, they had been just thirteen days away from being free . . . .

• • •

Although it technically is one, I don't think of this as a vegetarian cookbook. Eating healthfully is not about vegetarianism, veganism, or any other "-ism." From a nutrition standpoint, the reason I don't like the terms *vegetarian* and *vegan* is that they are defined by what you *don't* eat. Too often I meet vegans who proudly tell me about their animal-free diet . . . which seems to be composed primarily of french fries, fake meat, and nondairy ice cream. That

menu may be vegan, but it isn't particularly health-promoting.

This is why I prefer the term *whole-food, plant-based nutrition*. The best available balance of evidence suggests the healthiest diet is one that minimizes the intake of meat, eggs, dairy, and processed junk, and maximizes the intake of fruits, vegetables, legumes (beans, split peas, chickpeas, and lentils), whole grains, nuts and seeds, mushrooms, and herbs and spices—basically, real food that grows out of the ground. Those are our healthiest choices.

What do I mean by *whole food*? I mean a food that is not overly processed. In other words, nothing bad has been added, and nothing good has been taken away.

A classic example of food processing is the milling of grains, such as transforming whole wheat into white flour or "polishing" brown rice into white rice. White rice may have a clean look, but it's also practically devoid of the essential nutrients found in brown rice, such as B vitamins. Before food manufacturers started refortifying white rice with vitamins, millions of people died from beriberi, a vitamin B-deficiency disease that resulted from eating nutritionally empty white rice. Even though refined grains are now typically fortified with a few vitamins, they are still deficient in all the myriad phytonutrients found in the whole grain.

Using my definition of *nothing bad added, nothing good taken away*, I consider steel-cut oats, rolled oats, and even (plain) instant oatmeal relatively unprocessed, though the best option whenever possible is whole, intact grains.

By *plant-based*, I mean centering one's diet on as many whole plant foods as possible. For

How Not to Die, I created a traffic-light system to classify the Green Light foods people should eat more of, the Yellow Light foods we should eat less of, and the Red Light foods we should ideally avoid on a daily basis. It matters little what healthy folks eat on their birthday, holidays, and special occasions. It's the day-to-day stuff that adds up. As Kaiser Permanente's guide *The Plant-Based Diet: A Healthier Way to Eat* puts it: "If you find you cannot do a plant-based diet 100 percent of the time, then aim for 80 percent. Any movement toward more plants and fewer animal products [and processed foods] can improve your health!"[3]

I've tried to ensure all the recipes in this book are composed only of Green Light ingredients. This is not to say that all processed foods are bad for you. Foods are not so much good or bad as they are better or worse. Unprocessed foods tend to be more healthful than processed ones. Think of it this way: adding almonds to your oatmeal is better than putting almond milk on it, whereas almond milk would be better than putting dairy milk on it.

• • •

How Not to Die was inspired by my remarkable grandmother who was told at just sixty-five years old that her life was over. Her doctors sent her home in a wheelchair to die. However, soon after being discharged from the hospital, she was watching television and saw a *60 Minutes* segment about Nathan Pritikin, who was a pioneer in reversing heart disease through eating a plant-based diet. My grandmother flew to Pritikin's center in California to see whether his plan might help her. They wheeled her in, and she walked out on her own two feet, healthy. She was able to live thirty-one additional years beyond her death sentence—to continue to enjoy life with her six grandkids, including me.

This book was inspired by you, my readers and supporters, who have asked me so often about my favorite recipes, specific recommendations on meal planning, and the best ways to get as many of the Daily Dozen into your life as possible. I hope I can do for your family what Pritikin did for mine.

THE HOW NOT TO DIE APPROACH

For those of you who have not yet read or listened to *How Not to Die*, I encourage you to pick up a copy at your local bookstore or library. I have no personal financial stake in book sales. All the proceeds I receive from sales of any of my books, DVDs, and speaking engagements are donated to charity. So, it's not for personal gain that I hope you'll check out my last book. I truly believe it can help you live a healthier and happier life.

What follows here is a very brief summary of *How Not to Die*'s subject matter. This quick synopsis will help you understand the reason I've included these specific (and delicious) recipes in this companion cookbook—they all contain the whole plant foods that may be most helpful in warding off disease and restoring health.

• • •

In the late 1950s, forty-one-year-old engineer Nathan Pritikin was diagnosed with coronary heart disease. His doctors told him there was nothing he could do but take lots of naps, avoid stairs, and spend as much time as possible with his family. But instead of waiting for the inevitable, Pritikin took matters into his own hands and devoured everything he could find on his disease. His research eventually inspired him to adopt a plant-based diet, and within two years, his cholesterol plummeted from over 300 to below 160. Rather than dropping dead from a heart attack, Pritikin went on to help countless others reverse their own heart disease. One was my grandma who, as detailed in Pritikin's biography, became one of his most famous success stories.[4]

My grandmother's miraculous recovery is what inspired me to go to medical school. When I got there, however, I was shocked to find out this whole body of evidence on reversing chronic disease with lifestyle changes—opening up arteries without drugs or surgery—was largely being ignored by mainstream medicine. If effectively the *cure* to our leading cause of death could get lost down the rabbit hole and ignored, what other information might be buried in the medical literature? I made it my life's mission to find out. That's what led me to start NutritionFacts.org and that's what led me to write *How Not to Die*.

Plant-based nutrition is the only diet that's ever been proven to reverse heart disease in the majority of patients. If that's all a plant-based diet could do—reverse our number one killer—then shouldn't that be the default diet until proven otherwise? Even more so, since it can also be effective in treating, arresting, and reversing some of our other leading killers as well.

In *How Not to Die*, I cover the role diet may play in preventing and reversing each of the fifteen leading causes of premature death. Here they are, in order, starting with the most common condition, and the one my grandma was able to reverse so successfully.

CORONARY HEART DISEASE. Our number one killer lays waste to 375,000 Americans each year.[5] But, as the China-Cornell-Oxford Project suggested, it doesn't have to be that way. Led by Professor Emeritus T. Colin Campbell, this exhaustive study examined the dietary habits and mortality rates of several hundred thousand rural Chinese and later became the basis for Dr. Campbell's best-selling book *The China Study*. Amazingly, Campbell and colleagues found that many of our Western epidemics of chronic disease, including coronary heart disease, were absent among plant-based Chinese populations.[6] Similar studies conducted early in the twentieth century in rural Africa found the same thing: plant-based populations appeared to suffer one hundred times fewer heart attacks compared to Americans of the same age.[7]

Autopsies of accidental death victims have revealed that heart disease begins very early in life.[8] In fact, heart disease may even begin in the womb if your mother had high cholesterol.[9] In 1953, a study in the *Journal of the American Medical Association* examined three hundred fallen American soldiers from the Korean War, with an average age of twenty-two. The researchers found that 77 percent of the soldiers already had visible evidence of coronary atherosclerosis, and some even had arteries that were blocked off by 90 percent or more.[10] Other studies of accidental death victims have shown that fatty streaks—the precursor to plaque buildup—tend to appear by age ten among those eating the standard American diet.[11]

We couldn't be sure it was the food, though, until it was put to the test. Dr. Dean Ornish was the first to prove in a randomized controlled trial that a plant-based diet and other healthy lifestyle changes could reverse heart disease.[12] Dr. Caldwell Esselstyn Jr. followed up using just the dietary component. In 2014, he published a study involving nearly two hundred patients with severe heart disease—some like my grandma who couldn't make it to the mailbox without being crippled over in pain.

At the onset of the trial, Dr. Esselstyn told his patients to adopt a whole-food, plant-based diet. After making the switch, more than 99 percent of his compliant patients avoided further major cardiac events.[13]

LUNG DISEASES. Lung cancer, chronic obstructive pulmonary disease (COPD), and asthma collectively kill 296,000 Americans every year.[14] A plant-based diet may be able to help prevent all three. While the best way to prevent lung cancer is to avoid smoking, a single stalk of broccoli per day can boost the activity of detoxifying enzymes in the liver, helping to prevent lung-cancer–causing DNA damage at the cellular level.[15] Each daily serving of fruit is associated with men having a 24 percent lower risk of dying from COPD—a condition including emphysema that makes it difficult to breathe and gets worse over time. Finally, high vegetable consumption is associated with just half the odds of children developing asthma.[17] As far as treating asthma, simply adding a few more servings of fruits and vegetables to your diet has been shown in a randomized controlled trial to cut asthma attacks in half.[18]

BRAIN DISEASES. The two most serious brain diseases are stroke and Alzheimer's, which collectively kill 215,000 Americans each year.[19] Both have touched my life: my mom's father died of a stroke, and her mother of Alzheimer's. With most strokes, blood flow to the brain is cut off, depriving it of oxygen. The consequences wrought by a stroke depend on which area of the brain was damaged. People who experience a brief stroke might only need to contend with arm or leg weakness, whereas those who suffer a major stroke can be struck with paralysis, lose the ability to speak, or, as is too often the case, die.

Fortunately, a plant-based diet may reduce the odds of a stroke. Increasing intake of fiber (which is found only in plants) by only 7 grams per day—that's about a cup of raspberries—is associated with a 7 percent risk reduction.[20] In addition, a meta-analysis in the *Journal of the American College of Cardiology* found that increasing your potassium intake by 1,640 mg—a cup of cooked greens or a half-cup of beans—was associated with a 21 percent reduction in stroke risk.[21]

Alzheimer's, a horrendous disease that destroys our memory and sense of self, can neither be cured nor treated effectively. However, there is an emerging consensus that the same foods that clog our arteries can also clog our brain. A senior scientist at the Center for Alzheimer's Research entitled a review article "Alzheimer's Disease Is Incurable but Preventable."[22] Autopsies have shown repeatedly that Alzheimer's patients tend to have significantly more atherosclerotic plaque buildup and narrowing of the arteries within the brain.[23]

Numerous studies have shown that Alzheimer's is not a primarily genetic disease. For example, the Alzheimer's rates among Japanese men living in the United States are much higher than those of Japanese men living in Japan.[24] The same goes for African Americans in Indianapolis compared to Africans in Nigeria.[25] The problem may be the typical American diet, which can choke the arteries within the brain. Where is the world's lowest validated rate of Alzheimer's? Rural northern India,[26] where people traditionally eat a plant-based diet centered on grains and vegetables.[27]

DIGESTIVE CANCERS. Every year, 106,000 Americans die from cancers that might well have been prevented.[28] While some cancers have a significant genetic component, common digestive cancers are more likely the result of poor dietary choices. If you were to flatten out your intestines, they could cover thousands of square feet.[29] This means an extraordinary amount of surface area interacts with your food as it travels through your digestive tract. Food is our single greatest exposure to the outside environment. Colorectal (colon and rectal) cancer is one of the most commonly diagnosed cancers in the United States, but it's relatively rare in India. Comparatively, American men have eleven times more colorectal cancer diagnoses and women have ten times more.[30] One possible reason? Spices, such as turmeric, a staple of Indian cuisine, including curry powder, appear to have a variety of anticancer properties.[31] Another possibility is the food in which the turmeric-laden curry powder is used: India is one of the world's largest producers of fruits and vegetables, and only about 7 percent of the adult population eats meat on a daily basis. What most of this population does eat daily are legumes (beans, split peas, chickpeas, and lentils) and dark green, leafy vegetables,[32] which are packed with another class of cancer-fighting compounds called phytates.

Pancreatic cancer is among the most lethal cancers, with only 6 percent of patients surviving five years after diagnosis.[33] This is why prevention is paramount. The National Institutes of Health–AARP study, which followed 525,000 people aged fifty to seventy-one for years beginning in 1995, found the consumption of fat from animal sources was significantly associated with pancreatic cancer risk. No such correlation was found with consuming plant fats.[34] Likewise, the European Prospective Investigation into Cancer and Nutrition (EPIC) study, which followed 477,000 people for a decade beginning in 1992, found a 72 percent increased risk of pancreatic cancer for every 50 grams of poultry (about a quarter of a chicken breast) consumed daily.[35]

INFECTIONS. With each breath, we take in thousands of bacteria. With each bite of food comes millions more. Most microbes are harmless, but some cause serious infections, such as influenza and pneumonia, which alone kill fifty-seven thousand Americans each year.[36] A plant-based diet may be able to boost your immunity to keep you safer. In a 2012 study published in the *American Journal of Clinical Nutrition,* elderly volunteers who were randomized to eat five or more servings of fruit and vegetables daily had an 82 percent greater protective antibody response to a pneumonia vaccine compared to those who ate two or fewer servings a day.[37] In other words, you can bolster your immune system function just by eating more produce. Broccoli and other cruciferous vegetables have been shown to boost the effectiveness of intraepithelial lymphocytes, a special type of white blood cell that is the first line of gut defense against pathogens.[38] Blueberries, meanwhile, have been shown to almost double our levels of natural killer cells, which are vital members of the immune system's rapid response team against viruses and cancer cells.[39]

TYPE 2 DIABETES. More than twenty million Americans are currently diagnosed with diabetes, the "Black Death of the twenty-first century"—a tripling of cases since 1990.[40] Diabetes currently causes about 50,000 cases of kidney failure, 75,000 lower extremity amputations, 650,000 cases of vision loss, and about 75,000 deaths every year in the United States.[41] Type 2 diabetes is caused by our body's resistance to the effects of insulin, a vital hormone that shuttles glucose (blood sugar) into our cells, thereby preventing dangerous levels from accumulating in the blood. This insulin resistance is primarily caused by a fatty buildup inside our muscle cells.[42] This fat can come from excess fat in our diet or from excess fat on our body. Up to 90 percent of people who develop diabetes are overweight.[43]

A plant-based diet can help keep off the pounds. There appears to be a step-wise drop in obesity rates as one moves from nonvegetarian diets to flexitarian (part-time vegetarian) diets to pescatarian (fish-eating vegetarian) to vegetarian to vegan. Those eating strictly plant-based were the only dietary group that was on average at an ideal weight, with an average body mass index (BMI) of 23.6. (A BMI over 25 is considered overweight.) Nonvegetarians topped the charts at an unhealthy 28.8.[44] If you are trying to lose weight, including plant-based foods in your diet could help you: simply adding beans to diets was found to be as effective at slimming waistlines and improving blood sugar markers as calorie-cutting portion control.[45]

Based on a study of tens of thousands of adults in the United States and Canada, people who cut out all animal products, including fish, dairy, and eggs, appear to have a 78 percent reduced risk of diabetes.[46] If you already have diabetes, a plant-based diet may even reverse it. Even without weight loss, a plant-based diet can enable those who have had type 2 diabetes for decades get off all their insulin injections in as few as two weeks.[47] That's why if you're on medications to lower blood sugar or blood pressure, it's critical that you make these healthy changes under close medical supervision, so you can be rapidly weaned off these drugs if necessary. Otherwise the diet can work so well that your blood sugars or blood pressure can drop too low. Once your body has a chance to start healing itself, you can find yourself overmedicated very quickly.

HIGH BLOOD PRESSURE. Also known as hypertension, high blood pressure is the number one risk factor for death and disability worldwide,[48] laying waste to nine million people each year globally[49] and sixty-five thousand in the United States.[50] Increased blood pressure puts strain on your heart, can damage the sensitive blood vessels in your eyes and kidneys, and cause bleeding in the brain. Many doctors are under the impression that increased blood pressure is a natural consequence of aging, just like getting gray hair and wrinkles—after all, 65 percent of Americans over age sixty can expect to be diagnosed with hypertension.[51] But we've known for nearly a century that blood pressure can remain stable throughout life or actually decrease after age sixty.[52]

On average, high blood pressure medications reduce the risk of heart attack by 15 percent and the risk of stroke by about 25 percent.[53] But in a randomized, controlled trial, three portions of whole grains a day were able to help people achieve this same benefit without medication.[54] A cup of hibiscus herbal tea with each meal can lower systolic blood pressure by 6 points compared to a control group.[55] A double-blind, placebo-controlled, randomized trial found people with hypertension who consumed a few spoonfuls of flaxseeds every day for six months lowered their blood pressure on average from 158/82 to 143/75. That could be expected to result in 46 percent fewer strokes and 29 percent less heart disease over time.[56]

LIVER DISEASE. Many people assume that liver disease, which kills sixty thousand Americans each year,[57] is the result of heavy alcohol consumption or intravenous drug use. But nonalcoholic fatty liver disease (NAFLD) has quietly become the most common cause of chronic liver disease in the United States, afflicting an estimated seventy million people[58] and nearly 100 percent of those who are severely obese.[59] As with alcoholic fatty liver, NAFLD begins with the buildup of fat on the liver. In rare cases, this can cause inflammation and lead to fatal scarring of the liver, called cirrhosis.[60] Drinking just one can of soda per day appears to raise the odds of fatty liver disease by 45 percent.[61] People who eat the meat equivalent of fourteen chicken nuggets daily have nearly triple the rate of NAFLD compared to people who eat seven nuggets' worth or less.[62] One plant-based way to fight liver inflammation: Eating oatmeal was found in a double-blind, randomized, placebo-controlled trial to be able to significantly improve liver function among overweight men and women— and help them lose weight as well.[63]

BLOOD CANCERS. Leukemia, lymphoma, and multiple myeloma are sometimes referred to as liquid tumors because the cancer cells often circulate throughout the body rather than get concentrated in a solid mass. Every year these cancers kill fifty-six thousand Americans.[64] One of the largest studies on diet and cancer found that people who consume a more plant-based diet are less likely to develop all forms of cancer combined, with the greatest apparent protection against blood cancers.[65] The Iowa Women's Health Study, which has followed more than thirty-five thousand women for decades, showed that higher broccoli or other cruciferous vegetable intake was associated with a lower risk of non-Hodgkin's lymphoma.[66] This is consistent with a study at the Mayo Clinic that found people who ate about three or more servings of green, leafy vegetables per week appeared to have only about half the odds of getting lymphoma compared with those who ate less than one serving a week.[67] This protection may be due to the high antioxidant content of plant foods. It's important to note that this benefit is not found for antioxidant supplements.

KIDNEY DISEASE. Your kidneys filter 150 quarts of blood every twenty-four hours to produce the 1 to 2 quarts of urine you pee out each day. If the kidneys aren't functioning correctly, metabolic waste products can accumulate in the blood and eventually lead to dangerous problems, including weakness, shortness of breath, confusion, and abnormal heart rhythms. Eventually they can fail altogether, resulting in death unless regular dialysis is performed—a fate that befalls nearly forty-seven thousand Americans each year.[68]

A recent national survey found that only 41 percent of Americans tested had normal kidney function.[69] Most people with kidney disease may not even know they are suffering from it.[70] Researchers at Harvard University followed the diet and kidney function of thousands of healthy women for more than a decade. They concluded that three specific dietary components are associated with declining kidney function: animal protein, animal fat, and cholesterol.[71] Each is found only in one place: animal products.

Animal protein triggers an inflammatory reaction in the kidneys.[72] Within hours of your consuming meat, your kidneys rev up into hyperfiltration mode.[73] (*Hyperfiltration* means that your kidneys start to work overtime as increasing pressure builds up within them.) A lifetime of overeating animal protein may take its toll on your kidneys, causing them to be less and less efficient as you age. But your kidneys can handle the same amount of plant protein without a problem.[74] Plant protein may even help preserve function in ailing kidneys.[75]

BREAST CANCER. Killing forty thousand American women each year,[76] breast cancer is among the most feared diagnoses a woman can receive—and what we eat matters. The Long Island Breast Cancer Study Project found that postmenopausal women eating more grilled, barbecued, or smoked meats over their lifetime were associated with as much as 47 percent higher odds of breast cancer.[77] In the largest study on cholesterol and cancer to date—with more than a million participants—a 17 percent increased breast cancer risk was found in premenopausal women who had total cholesterol levels over 240 compared with women whose cholesterol was under 160.[78] This means that the same plant-based diet that helps lower a woman's risk of heart disease may also help lower her risk of breast cancer. The Black Women's Health Study, which followed fifty thousand African American women beginning in 1995, found that women who ate two or more servings of vegetables a day had a significantly decreased risk of a kind of breast cancer that's hard to treat: estrogen-receptor-negative and progesterone-receptor-negative.[79] In premenopausal women, a high-fiber diet was associated with an extraordinary 85 percent lower odds of that type of estrogen-receptor-negative breast tumors.[80]

SUICIDAL DEPRESSION. Forty-one thousand Americans take their life every year,[81] and depression is a leading cause.[82] While anyone experiencing suicidal thoughts should seek professional help, lifestyle interventions can help heal the mind as well as the body. One way to fight the blues may be with greens: higher consumption of vegetables may cut the odds of developing depression by as much as 62 percent.[83] In general, eating lots of fruits and veggies may present "a non-invasive, natural, and inexpensive therapeutic means to support a healthy brain."[84] Additionally, the spice saffron was found to be as effective at treating mild to moderate depression as the antidepressant drug Prozac[85]—and it tastes a lot better.

PROSTATE CANCER. Prostate cancer is much more common than most people think: autopsy studies have shown that about half of men over the age of eighty suffer from it.[86] Most die of other diseases first, but prostate cancer still kills twenty-eight thousand men every year.[87] Recent studies have revealed a link between diet and prostate cancer. Population studies have suggested the prevalence of prostate cancer increases as animal consumption increases. For example, the death rate of prostate cancer in Japan has increased twenty-five-fold since World War II, and this dramatic spike coincides with a twenty-fold increase in dairy consumption, a seven-fold increase in egg consumption, and a nine-fold increase in meat consumption.[88] Dairy consumption has been consistently associated with risk: a 2015 meta-analysis and review found that high intakes of dairy products—milk and cheese (including low- and nonfat varieties) but not nondairy sources of calcium—appear to increase total prostate cancer risk.[89]

If you have early-stage prostate cancer, you may be able to reverse its progression with a plant-based diet. After conquering our number-one killer, heart disease, Dr. Dean Ornish moved on to killer number two, cancer. Prostate cancer patients were randomized into two groups: a control group that wasn't given any diet or lifestyle advice beyond whatever their personal doctors told them to do, and a healthy-living group prescribed a plant-based diet centered on fruits, vegetables, whole grains, and beans, along with other healthy lifestyle behaviors. After a year, the control group's blood PSA—a marker of prostate cancer growth inside the body—tended to increase, but the plant-based group's PSA levels tended to go down,[90] which suggests their prostate tumors actually shrank. No surgery, no chemotherapy, no radiation—just eating and living healthily.

PARKINSON'S DISEASE. A disease of prizefighters and NFL linebackers who sustain repeated head trauma, Parkinson's disease, which kills twenty-five thousand Americans every year,[91] may also be due to brain damage caused by exposure to pollutants and toxic heavy metals that build up in the food supply. Poultry and tuna have been found to be the leading food sources of arsenic; dairy, the number one source of lead; and seafood, including tuna, the number one source of mercury.[92] An analysis of more than twelve thousand food and feed samples across twenty countries found that the highest contamination of the toxic chemical polychlorinated biphenyl (PCB) was found in fish and fish oil, followed by eggs, dairy, and then other meats. The lowest contamination was found at the bottom of the food chain, in plants.[93] Those who eat a plant-based diet have been found to have significantly lower blood levels of a PCB implicated in increasing the risk of developing Parkinson's disease.[94]

Wait a minute, Doc, some of you eagle-eyed readers might be thinking. *That's only fourteen.* Indeed! The fifteenth killer is actually the third-leading cause of death, responsible for 225,000 deaths annually.[95] Oh, and it's not a disease.

It's doctors.

That's right. Medical care is the third-leading cause of death. Whether it's death caused by a hospital infection,[96] unnecessary surgery, receiving the wrong medication, or an adverse side effect from the right medication,[97] the sad reality is that you can head into a routine procedure and never return home. While hospitals are striving to reduce medical error and the spread of infections, they remain dangerous places.[98] Did you know that getting a routine chest CT scan is estimated to inflict the same cancer risk as smoking seven hundred cigarettes?[99] Or that 1 middle-aged woman in every 270 may develop cancer after a single CT angiogram?[100] Or that when it comes to cholesterol, blood pressure, and blood-thinning drugs, the chance of even high-risk patients benefiting from them is typically less than 5 percent over a period of five years?[101] Doctors and patients alike wildly overestimate the power of pills and procedures to ward off death and disability.

To me, the true tragedy is all the lost opportunities to address the root causes of chronic disease. Our modern medical system is great at fixing broken bones and curing infections, but it fails woefully at preventing and reversing the most common causes of death. Until the system changes, we have to take personal responsibility for our own health and our family's. We can't wait until society catches up to the science, because it's a matter of life and death. I wrote *How Not to Die* to help you understand the role foods can play in preventing, arresting, or reversing the fifteen leading causes of death. I wrote this book to help you actually do it, right in your own kitchen.

THE DAILY DOZEN

Many have told me *How Not to Die* is their nutrition "bible."

I've been honored to hear from countless laypeople who've shared their enthusiasm for *How Not to Die*, and high school students to graduate students—even professors—have told me they've used it as their go-to source for papers and lectures. Yes, I cite thousands of peer-reviewed papers from the scientific literature, but I didn't want to just write a reference book. I also wanted to create a practical guide on translating this mountain of evidence into easy-to-make, day-to-day decisions, and that's how I shaped the second half of the book. I center my recommendations around a Daily Dozen checklist of all the things I try to fit into my daily routine and encourage you to, as well.

And, yes: There's an app for that. "Dr. Greger's Daily Dozen" is available as a free app for Android and iPhone. The app specifies serving sizes and can help you keep track of how you're doing.

For my family, the Daily Dozen checklist has been a useful reminder to try to make each meal as healthful as possible. I was so heartened to find out that others found it helpful, too. I've gotten literally thousands of emails from people who excitedly tell me how many check marks they're up to that day.

"I eat more cruciferous vegetables than I ever thought possible," one woman told me, "and I never even knew the word *cruciferous* before!" Other people say that ground flaxseeds are now such a basic part of their life that they pack a containerful when they travel. Others tell me they'd never cooked with spices until they read the book, but now that they do, they not only reap the health benefits of turmeric, oregano, and the rest, but also find that their meals taste better than ever.

Lots of people have made it into a game. To get in all the servings I recommend, you have to tick off 24 checkboxes a day. People kept asking for meal plans and recipes to help them nail the Daily Dozen every day. I love hearing about all the creative ways readers have told me they are trying to incorporate things like beans and greens into breakfast, but many were left wondering how to shop for, prepare, and serve them. What they wanted, they said, was a cookbook.

So, here it is: *The How Not to Die Cookbook*. Its purpose is to give you recipes for meals that are delicious, nutritious, and, of course, help you include all of the Daily Dozen in your life as often as possible.

Centering your diet on the Daily Dozen should make it easier to stay healthy. Remember, eating is a zero-sum game. When you decide to eat one food, it means you are choosing not to eat another food. After all, there's only so much you can consume in one day. So, whatever you choose has an opportunity cost.

That means every time you put something in your mouth, it's a lost opportunity to invest in something healthier. Think of it this way: If you had $2,000 in the bank to spend on food, how would you want to use it? Would you lavish it on wonderful meals that let you check off most of the items on the Daily Dozen list? Or would you waste it on buckets of fried chicken and bags of Cheetos? I'd like to think that if you've picked up this book, you'd choose the former. In reality, you only have about 2,000 calories to "spend" each day, and each food choice determines whether you are spending them on something that enriches your health, or bankrupts it.

The recipes in this book will give you the opportunity to prepare meals that provide you with the most nutritional bang for your caloric buck. From Mango-Avocado-Kale Salad with Ginger-Sesame Orange Dressing to Black Bean Soup with Quinoa & Kale to Stuffed Portobellos with Herbed Mushroom Gravy, you will find recipes that make your mouth water and keep your body healthy.

NOTE: *The Daily Dozen represents the twelve things I try to make part of my day, every day. This means anything from five servings of a healthy beverage to at least one serving each of berries, flaxseeds, nuts and seeds, and herbs and spices. You will see a list at the end of each recipe telling you which of the Daily Dozen each recipe includes.*

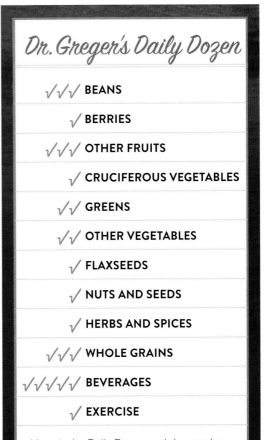

Here is the Daily Dozen and the number of servings I recommend for each one. For years, I had this list on a little dry-erase board on our refrigerator. Feel free to cut this one out (or make your own copy) and do the same. It's also useful to take with you when you go shopping to guide you through your healthiest choices. And remember, it's just about doing your best. There are times, especially when I am traveling, that I only hit a quarter of my goals. When that happens, I just try to make up for it the next day. The same goes for you: if one day you only get a few of these foods into your diet, the next day, do your best to get more!

ONE

SIMPLE PREPARATIONS

Before we dive into the incredible recipes we've created for you, I wanted to first share ten flavor-makers that you'll use in many of the recipes throughout the book. I love them all, but two of my favorites are Savory Spice Blend, a seasoning mix that not only adds enormous zest, but is salt-free, and Umami Sauce, another flavor enhancer that is a delicious alternative to soy sauce preparations such as stir-fries and sautés. Also in this chapter are recipes for making your own almond milk and vegetable broth, a healthy version of Parmesan cheese to sprinkle on pasta dishes, date syrup, balsamic glaze, and ranch dressing, as well as simple instructions on how to roast garlic.

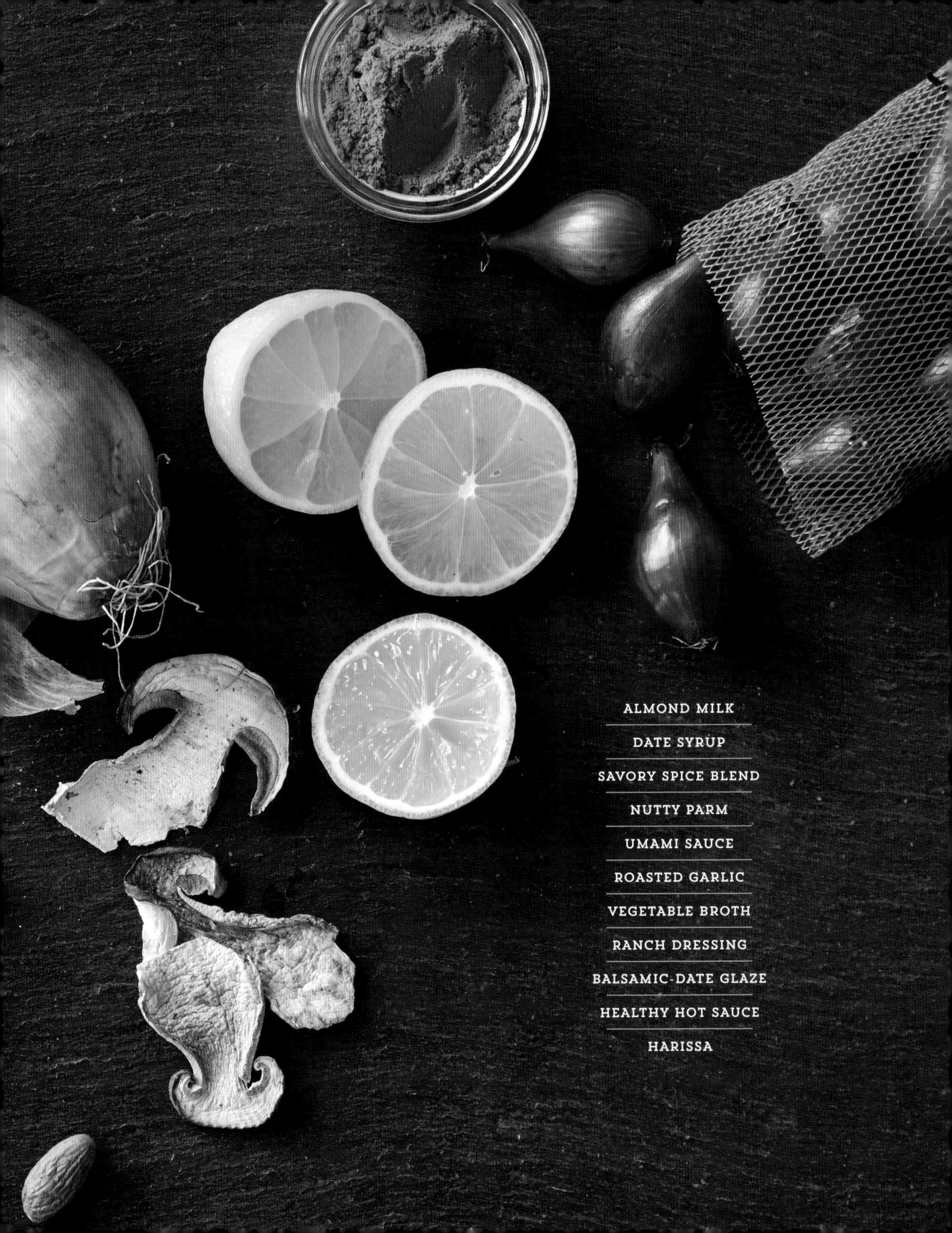

ALMOND MILK

DATE SYRUP

SAVORY SPICE BLEND

NUTTY PARM

UMAMI SAUCE

ROASTED GARLIC

VEGETABLE BROTH

RANCH DRESSING

BALSAMIC-DATE GLAZE

HEALTHY HOT SAUCE

HARISSA

- If using dried beans, cook them in large batches and then portion and freeze them. I used to use canned beans until I discovered how easy it is to prepare dried beans from scratch, using an electric pressure cooker.

- Instead of making one or two servings at a time, cook a large pot of a staple grain or a grain with a quick-cooking legume, such as lentils, mixed in. Then, simply portion and freeze until you want to thaw, heat, and enjoy.

- Prepare double batches of recipes for long-cooking dishes, such as stews, soups, or chilies. You'll not only save time—you'll get more enhanced flavor when you reheat. They're even better when served later in the week or after being frozen for a time.

- Make seasoning blends, sauces, or dressings ahead of time to have on hand.

- Double up on prep, such as chopping onions, when making more than one recipe, so you have enough for both. When you only need half an onion, chop the whole onion and refrigerate the unused portion in a sealed container.

TRAFFIC LIGHT SYSTEM

In *How Not to Die*, I explain what I call Dining by Traffic Light. This is a system that is as easy to follow as obeying a traffic light. Green is for go. Green Light foods, which are unprocessed plant foods, should make up the bulk of our diet. Yellow is for caution. Yellow Light foods include processed plant foods and unprocessed animal foods. Red is for stop, as in stop and think before you put it in your mouth. Red Light foods are the ultraprocessed plant foods and processed animal foods. The more green lights you hit, the faster you'll get to your health destination!

ALMOND MILK

MAKES: ABOUT *2* CUPS · DIFFICULTY: *easy*

Here's a fast and easy way to make a whole-food almond milk. For taste and convenience I personally prefer unsweetened soy milk. (I like the flavor of Whole Foods Market's store brand the best.) But I wanted to embrace the challenge of creating recipes containing only Green Light ingredients. This doesn't offer the calcium, vitamin D, and B12 fortification of commercial almond milks, but it avoids the added salt and thickeners of questionable safety, such as carrageenan. Choose almond butter made from raw rather than roasted or toasted almonds to decrease exposure to advanced glycation end products. (See page 108.)

2 tablespoons smooth raw almond butter

2 cups water

Combine the almond butter and water in a high-speed blender and blend until smooth. Transfer the milk to a glass bottle or jar with a tight-fitting lid and chill until ready to serve. Shake well before using.

DATE SYRUP

MAKES: ABOUT *1½* CUPS · DIFFICULTY: *easy*

Green Light sweeteners are a little hard to come by. Date sugar, which is simply dried, pulverized dates, can be used as a whole-food, granulated sugar, and blackstrap molasses is a good choice for a healthy liquid sweetener, but it has a strong, sometimes overpowering flavor. We've come up with our own DIY date syrup we hope you'll love as much as we do.

1 cup pitted dates

1 cup boiling water

1 teaspoon blended peeled lemon (see sidebar)

Combine the dates and hot water in a heatproof bowl and set aside for 1 hour to soften the dates. Transfer the dates and water to a high-speed blender. Add the lemon and blend until smooth. Transfer to a glass jar or other airtight container with a tight-fitting lid. Store the syrup in the refrigerator for up to 2 to 3 weeks.

USING BLENDED WHOLE LEMONS AND LIMES

Instead of cooking with lemon or lime juice, use the blended whole fruit to get more nutritional benefit. When you use just the juice, you lose out on the fiber and all the nutrition that was attached to it.

Here's a great time-saver when cooking with blended lemon or lime. Peel and blend a whole lemon and then freeze it in 1-teaspoon portions—a small silicone ice cube tray is ideal for this. Then, grab a cube from the freezer whenever you need it!

SAVORY SPICE BLEND

MAKES: ABOUT ½ CUP · DIFFICULTY: *easy*

I always have this seasoning blend on hand to add flavor to dishes in place of salt.

---

2 tablespoons nutritional yeast*

1 tablespoon onion powder

1 tablespoon dried parsley

1 tablespoon dried basil

2 teaspoons dried thyme

2 teaspoons garlic powder

2 teaspoons dry mustard (mustard powder)

2 teaspoons paprika

½ teaspoon ground turmeric

½ teaspoon celery seeds

Combine all the ingredients in a spice grinder or blender to mix well and pulverize the dried herbs and spices. Transfer the blend to a shaker bottle or jar with a tight-fitting lid. Store in a cool, dry place.

* *I recommend those with Crohn's disease or hidradenitis suppurativa avoid nutritional yeast.*

NUTTY PARM

MAKES: ABOUT 1½ CUPS · DIFFICULTY: *easy*

For a cheesy flavor, sprinkle this on pasta, grain dishes, salads, and snacks like popcorn or kale chips.

½ cup almonds

½ cup Brazil nuts

½ cup nutritional yeast*

2 teaspoons Savory Spice Blend (page 4)

Combine all the ingredients in a food processor and process until the nuts are finely ground. Transfer to a covered container or shaker and keep refrigerated.

VARIATION: Substitute different nuts for the almonds or Brazil nuts.

UMAMI SAUCE

MAKES: ABOUT *1¼* CUPS · DIFFICULTY: *easy*

Use this sauce in sautés or stir-fries to boost flavor without adding all the sodium of soy sauce. Umami is one of the five basic tastes, even though many people are only learning about it now. This word was created by a Japanese chemist named Kikunae Ikeda from *umai*, which means "delicious," and *mi*, which means "taste." The perfect name, as it is a delicious taste!

1 cup Vegetable Broth (page 6)

1 teaspoon minced garlic

1 teaspoon grated fresh ginger

1 tablespoon blackstrap molasses

1½ teaspoons Date Syrup (page 3) or date sugar

½ teaspoon jarred tomato paste

½ teaspoon ground black pepper

1½ teaspoons white miso paste blended with 2 tablespoons water

2 teaspoons blended peeled lemon (see page 3)

1 tablespoon rice vinegar*

Heat the broth in a small saucepan over medium heat. Add the garlic and ginger and simmer for 3 minutes. Stir in the molasses, Date Syrup, tomato paste, and black pepper and bring just to a boil. Reduce the heat to low and simmer for 1 minute. Remove from the heat, and then stir in the miso mixture, blended lemon, and rice vinegar. Taste and adjust the seasonings, if needed. Allow the sauce to cool before transferring to a jar or bottle with a tight-fitting lid or pouring the sauce into an ice cube tray and freezing into individual portions.

* *Vinegar is an honorary Green Light condiment because of the health-promoting benefits of its acetic acid.*

ROASTED GARLIC

MAKES: ABOUT *3* TABLESPOONS (PER HEAD OF GARLIC) · DIFFICULTY: *easy*

Easy to prepare, roasted garlic adds incredible bursts of flavor to recipes and makes a great spread on toast or sandwiches.

---

1 whole head garlic, or more

Preheat the oven to 400°F. Use a sharp knife to cut about ⅓ inch off the top of a whole garlic head to expose the tops of the garlic cloves. Wrap the garlic head in parchment paper or place in a small covered baking dish, cut side up, and place in the oven. If roasting more than one head of garlic, arrange them, cut side up, in a covered baking dish, or place each head in a separate well of a muffin pan and cover with an inverted cookie sheet. Bake for 35 to 45 minutes, or until the garlic cloves are soft and golden brown. Remove from the oven and uncover to let the garlic cool. When the garlic is cool to the touch, gently squeeze each clove individually over a small bowl, allowing the soft, roasted garlic to slip out of the papery skin. (If it is not very soft and golden brown, it needs to be covered or rewrapped in the parchment and baked a few minutes longer.) Enjoy the roasted garlic immediately or store it in the refrigerator in a jar or other container with a tight-fitting lid.

VEGETABLE BROTH

MAKES: ABOUT *6* CUPS · DIFFICULTY: *easy*

Use this in any of the recipes calling for salt-free vegetable broth.

---

1 medium onion, coarsely chopped

1 carrot, cut into 1-inch pieces

2 celery ribs, coarsely chopped

3 garlic cloves, crushed

2 dried mushrooms

⅓ cup coarsely chopped fresh parsley

½ teaspoon ground black pepper

2 tablespoons white miso paste

Savory Spice Blend (page 4)

In a large pot, heat 1 cup of water over medium heat. Add the onion, carrot, celery, and garlic and cook for 5 minutes. Stir in the mushrooms, parsley, and black pepper. Add 7 cups of water and bring to a boil. Reduce the heat to low and simmer for 1½ hours. Let cool slightly and then transfer to a high-speed blender and blend until smooth. Return the blended broth back to the pot. Ladle about ⅓ cup of the broth into a small bowl or cup. Add the miso paste and stir well before incorporating into the broth. Add the Savory Spice Blend to taste. Let the broth cool to room temperature; then divide among containers with tight-sealing lids and store in the refrigerator or freezer. Properly stored, the stock will keep for up to 5 days in the refrigerator or up to 3 months in the freezer.

NOTE: If you don't have time to make your own broth, you can buy salt-free vegetable broth or salt-free vegetable bouillon cubes, available in natural food stores or online.

RANCH DRESSING

MAKES: ABOUT *1½* CUPS · DIFFICULTY: *easy*

Creamy and flavorful, this dressing isn't just for salads. Serve it as a dipping sauce for the Buffalo Cauliflower (page 183), crudités, or anything else you want to kick up a notch.

½ cup raw cashews, soaked for 3 hours and drained

2 cloves Roasted Garlic (page 6)

½ cup Almond Milk (page 2)

2 tablespoons rice vinegar

2 teaspoons blended peeled lemon (see page 3)

1 tablespoon chopped red onion

2 teaspoons Savory Spice Blend (page 4)

1 teaspoon white miso paste

¾ teaspoon date sugar

1 tablespoon minced fresh parsley

1 teaspoon chopped fresh dill, or ½ teaspoon dried

In a high-speed blender, combine all the ingredients except the parsley and dill, and blend until smooth. Transfer the dressing to a bowl and stir in the parsley and dill. Taste and adjust the seasonings, if needed. (The flavor will get stronger as the dressing sits.) Cover and refrigerate for at least an hour to allow the flavors to develop. Stir or shake before serving.

BALSAMIC-DATE GLAZE

MAKES: ABOUT *1* CUP · DIFFICULTY: *easy*

Drizzle this rich sauce over Stuffed Sweet Potatoes (page 176), your favorite roasted vegetables or grain dishes, salads, and fruits, such as watermelon or strawberries.

½ cup pitted dates

¾ cup warm water

½ cup balsamic vinegar

Soften the dates by soaking in warm water for about 10 minutes. In a blender, combine the dates and their soaking water with the balsamic vinegar. Blend until smooth.

Transfer the mixture to a small saucepan and bring to a boil; then reduce the heat to low. Simmer on low until the glaze is reduced and thickened, stirring frequently.

DATES

Growing up, I never liked dates. I thought they were dry and kind of waxy. But then I discovered there were soft, plump, moist varieties that didn't taste like the chalky ones I remembered. Bahri dates—my favorite—are wet and sticky, and when frozen, acquire the taste and chew of caramel candy. Dates are healthy, too: a 2009 study found that eating four to five dried dates per day may improve the antioxidant power of your bloodstream while bringing down triglyceride levels.[103]

HEALTHY HOT SAUCE

MAKES: ABOUT *2* CUPS · DIFFICULTY: *easy*

Most bottled hot sauces contain too much sodium. The good news is, it's easy to make your own—and you can leave out the salt!

12 ounces fresh hot chilies (a single type or mixed), stemmed, halved lengthwise, seeded, and chopped

½ cup chopped onion

1 tablespoon minced garlic

½ to 1 cup apple cider vinegar

In a saucepan, combine the chilies, onion, garlic, and ¼ cup of water over high heat. Cook, stirring, for 2 to 3 minutes. Lower the heat to medium-high, add 1¾ cups of water and continue to cook, stirring occasionally, for 15 to 20 minutes, or until the chilies are very soft. Remove from the heat and let the mixture come to room temperature.

Transfer the chili mixture to a food processor and process until very smooth. Add ½ cup of the vinegar and process to blend. Taste the sauce and add more of the vinegar, if desired, to taste. Transfer the hot sauce to a clean glass jar or bottle and secure with an airtight lid. Keep refrigerated. Can be stored in the refrigerator for up to 6 months.

NOTE: Be sure to use rubber gloves when handling hot chilies and do not touch your eyes.

HARISSA

MAKES: ABOUT *1½* CUPS · DIFFICULTY: *easy*

Harissa is an aromatic, spicy paste frequently used in North African and Middle Eastern cooking. It's usually made of hot chili peppers, garlic, olive oil, and such spices as caraway, coriander, cumin, and saffron—but these vary according to preference. Harissa is called the national condiment of Tunisia, where it seems most meals contain it. In the United States, you can find less-than-healthy versions at many markets in cans or tubes, which is why I've included a recipe here for you to enjoy.

⅓ cup dried hot red chilies, seeded and cut into small pieces, or to taste

1 tablespoon coriander seeds

2 teaspoons caraway seeds

1 teaspoon cumin seeds

2 roasted red bell peppers (see above, or store-bought)

3 garlic cloves, chopped

1 tablespoon nutritional yeast

2 teaspoons white miso paste

Savory Spice Blend (page 4)

Place the dried chilies in a heatproof bowl and cover with boiling water. Set aside for 30 minutes; then drain.

In a small skillet, stir the coriander, caraway, and cumin seeds over low heat until fragrant, about 30 seconds. Transfer to a food processor and add the drained chilies, roasted red bell peppers, garlic, nutritional yeast, miso, and Savory Spice Blend to taste. Process until smooth. Add up to ¼ cup of water, as needed, to make a smooth, thick sauce.

ROASTING RED BELL PEPPERS

Roast bell peppers by holding them directly over a gas flame with a pair of tongs until the skin blackens on all sides. They can also be roasted under a broiler, turning until the skin blackens all over. Place the blackened peppers in a bowl and cover tightly. Set aside for 10 minutes, or until cool enough to touch with your hands; then remove the blackened skin and the seeds and proceed with the recipe. If you'd rather not roast your own peppers, you can purchase jars of roasted red bell peppers in supermarkets.

TWO

BREAKFAST

This chapter offers many ways to start your day on the right foot—
even on those days when you get up on the wrong side of the bed.
I like to make whole grains part of my morning routine, whether it's with
oatmeal (with berries or chocolate) or Morning Grain Bowls. When I sit
down with my family, some of our favorite breakfast go-tos are
French Toast with Berry Drizzle, Burrito Breakfast Bake, and
Skillet Sweet Potato Hash. (If you're looking for smoothies,
you'll find them in the Sips chapter starting on page 204.)

SUMMERTIME OATMEAL

SUPERFOOD BREAKFAST BITES

FRENCH TOAST WITH BERRY DRIZZLE

WARM PEAR COMPOTE

CHOCOLATE OATMEAL

MORNING GRAIN BOWLS

BURRITO BREAKFAST BAKE

SKILLET SWEET POTATO HASH

SUMMERTIME OATMEAL

MAKES: *2* (1¼-CUP) SERVINGS · DIFFICULTY: *easy*

Some people think of oats as a hot cereal perfect for when leaves start falling or there's snow on the ground, but I love them all year round. In our house, we call this version Summertime Oatmeal because it's a cool and refreshing way to enjoy oatmeal even when it's sweltering outside. Prepare it the night before and spoon the goodness into jars for a quick and easy breakfast.

1 cup old-fashioned rolled oats

1 tablespoon chia seeds

1 tablespoon ground flaxseeds

½ teaspoon ground cinnamon

1¾ cups Almond Milk (page 2)

2 tablespoons Date Syrup (page 3)

1 2- to 3-inch piece vanilla bean, split and scraped (or 1 teaspoon extract)

⅔ cup fresh or frozen blueberries or strawberries

Combine all the ingredients in a medium bowl and stir to mix. Spoon into two 1-pint jars with tight-fitting lids or two small bowls and cover tightly. Refrigerate overnight and remove the vanilla bean before serving.

MAXIMIZING YOUR MORNING

Want to start your day with a five–check mark breakfast? Add berries, flaxseeds, nuts, and spices to your oatmeal. How about a six-plus–check mark smoothie? Create a thirst-quenching beverage by blending berries and other fruits, greens, flaxseeds, and spices. (See pages 210 and 216.)

Daily Dozen Foods

✗ BERRIES   ✗ OTHER FRUITS   ✗ NUTS AND SEEDS   ✗ WHOLE GRAINS

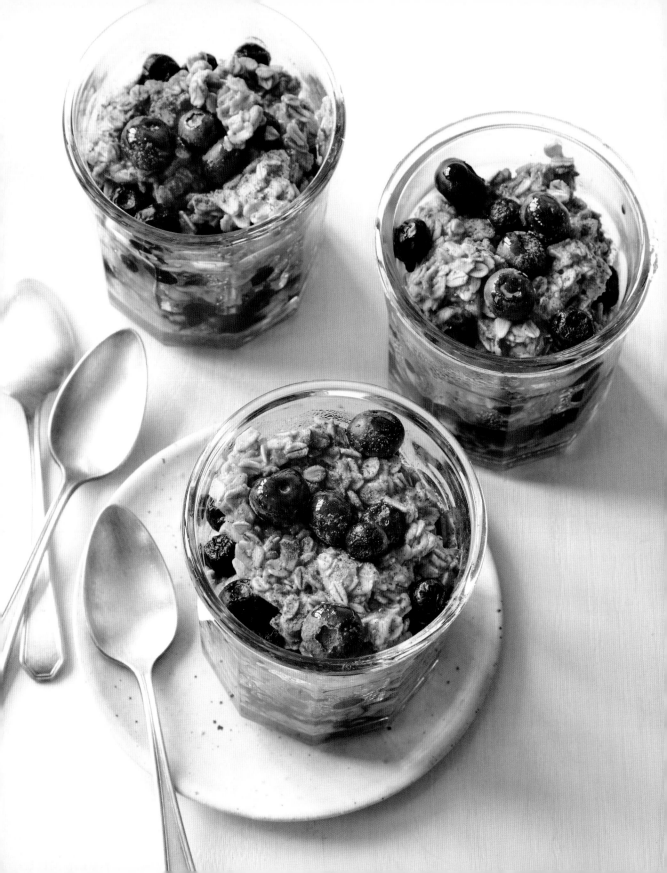

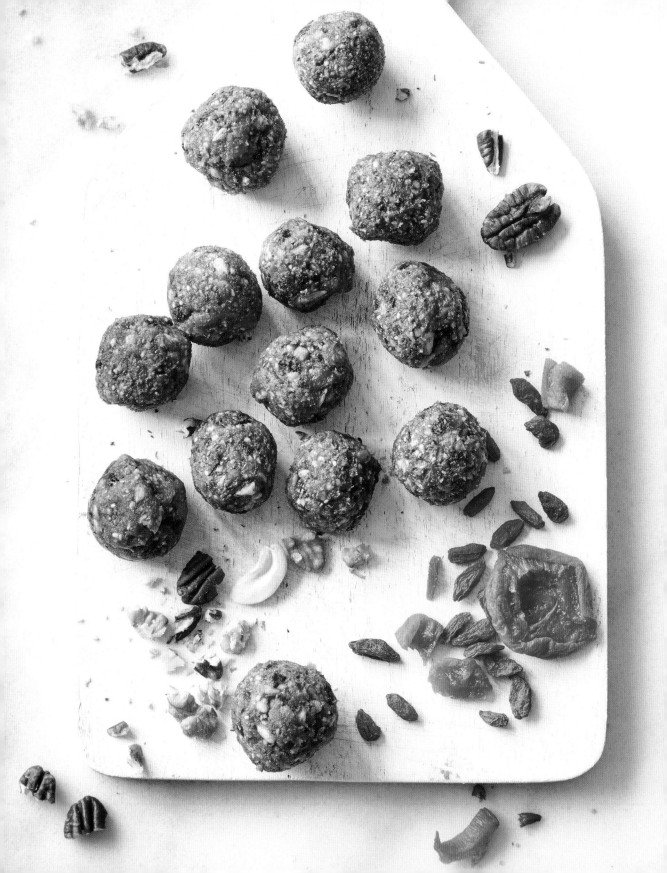

SUPERFOOD BREAKFAST BITES

MAKES: *24* (1-INCH) BITES (4 TO 6 SERVINGS) · DIFFICULTY: *easy*

Stash these delicious bites in the fridge for an easy on-the-go breakfast or after-workout snack.

¾ cup pitted dates, soaked in hot water for 20 minutes, then drained

¾ cup raw walnuts, pecans, or cashews

¾ cup dried cranberries, apricots, apple slices, or other dried fruit, chopped if necessary

¼ cup sunflower seeds

2 tablespoons goji berries or barberries

2 tablespoons chia seeds or hemp hearts (hulled hemp seeds)

2 tablespoons ground flaxseeds

1 1- to 1½-inch piece vanilla bean, split and scraped (or ½ teaspoon extract)

¼ teaspoon ground cinnamon

In a food processor, combine the drained dates and nuts and pulse until the nuts are finely ground and the dates are incorporated. Add the remaining ingredients and process until well combined. The mixture should be very sticky. If it seems too dry to hold together, add a little water, 1 tablespoon at a time. If the mixture is too wet, add a little more ground flaxseeds or some rolled oats.

Roll a heaping tablespoonful of the mixture between the palms of your hands to form a 1-inch ball. Transfer to a plate. Repeat until all the mixture has been rolled into balls. Cover the plate with foil or parchment paper and refrigerate for 4 hours before enjoying. Store in the refrigerator.

FLAXSEEDS

According to one remarkable study, flaxseeds "induced one of the most potent blood-pressure-lowering effects ever achieved by a dietary intervention."[104] Eating just a few tablespoons a day appears to be two to three times more effective at lowering blood pressure than adopting an aerobic endurance exercise program[105] (not that you shouldn't do both!). Another study found that sprinkling a few spoonfuls of ground flaxseeds on your meals may reduce the risk of breast cancer.[106]

Daily Dozen Foods

X BERRIES   X OTHER FRUITS   X FLAXSEEDS   X NUTS AND SEEDS   X HERBS AND SPICES

FRENCH TOAST
WITH BERRY DRIZZLE

MAKES: *4* SERVINGS · DIFFICULTY: *easy*

The turmeric gives a warm golden color to this festive breakfast that packs six of the Daily Dozen in one dish.

BERRY DRIZZLE

1 cup fresh or thawed frozen berries of choice

1 to 2 tablespoons Date Syrup (page 3)

FRENCH TOAST

1¼ cups Almond Milk (page 2)

2 tablespoons ground flaxseeds blended with ¼ cup warm water

1 tablespoon date sugar

1 1- to 1½-inch piece vanilla bean, split and scraped (or ½ teaspoon extract)

1 ¼-inch piece fresh turmeric, grated (or ¼ teaspoon ground)

¼ teaspoon ground cinnamon

8 slices salt-free 100% whole-grain bread

BERRY DRIZZLE: Combine the berries and Date Syrup in a blender and blend until smooth. Transfer to a small pitcher or bowl and set aside.

FRENCH TOAST: In a blender, combine the Almond Milk, flax mixture, date sugar, vanilla, turmeric, and cinnamon. Blend until well mixed. Transfer the batter to a shallow bowl. Heat a nonstick skillet or griddle over medium-high heat. Working in batches, dip the bread slices into the batter, coating both sides, then place in the hot skillet, and cook until golden brown on each side, turning once. Keep the cooked French toast warm in the oven set to its lowest temperature while you finish cooking the rest. When ready to serve, arrange the French toast on plates and drizzle with the berry syrup.

Daily Dozen Foods

✗ BERRIES   ✗ OTHER FRUITS   ✗ FLAXSEEDS   ✗ NUTS AND SEEDS   ✗ HERBS AND SPICES   ✗ WHOLE GRAINS

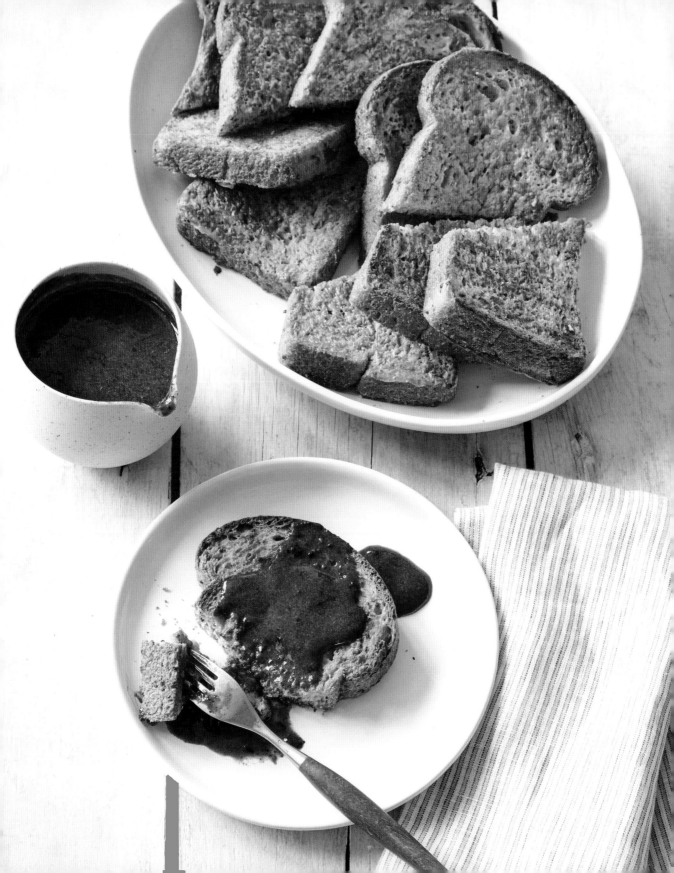

WARM PEAR COMPOTE

MAKES: *4* (½-CUP) SERVINGS · DIFFICULTY: *easy*

This delightful compote is a savory dessert or snack, as well as an incredible topping for oatmeal, French toast, or pancakes.

2 tablespoons date sugar

2 teaspoons blended peeled lemon (see page 3)

2 tablespoons raisins

1 2- to 3-inch piece vanilla bean, split and scraped (or 1 teaspoon extract)

1 teaspoon ground cinnamon

¼ teaspoon ground ginger

⅛ teaspoon ground nutmeg

1-inch piece fresh turmeric, grated (or ⅛ teaspoon ground)

4 to 5 ripe Bartlett pears, cored and cut into bite-sized pieces

In a saucepan, combine ½ cup of water with all the ingredients, except the pears, and stir. Once blended, add the pear pieces and simmer over low heat until the pears are tender and the sauce has reduced, 15 to 20 minutes. Serve warm.

VARIATION: Use chopped apples, peaches, or plums instead of pears.

Daily Dozen Foods

✗ OTHER FRUITS   ✗ HERBS AND SPICES

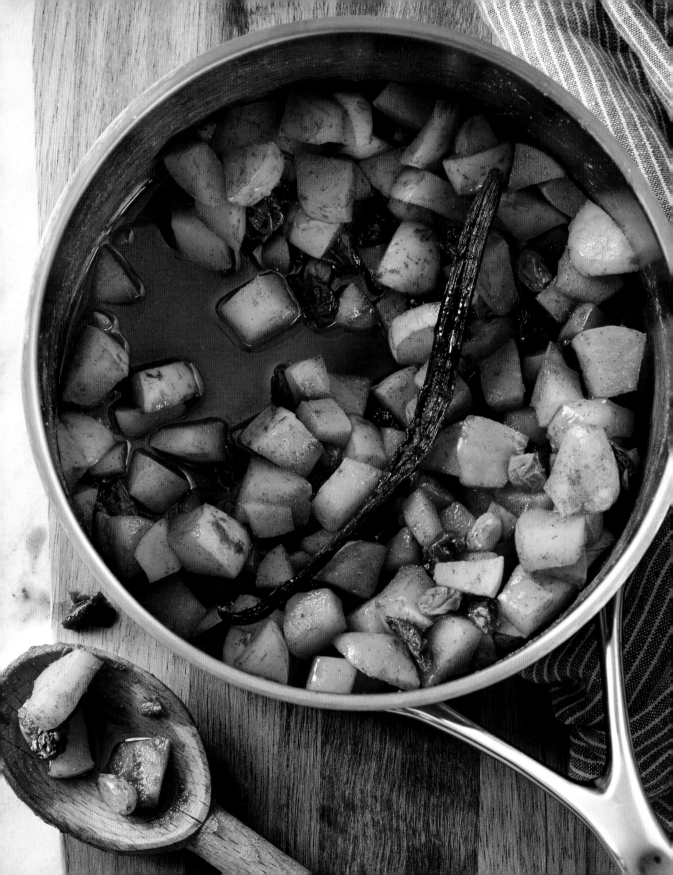

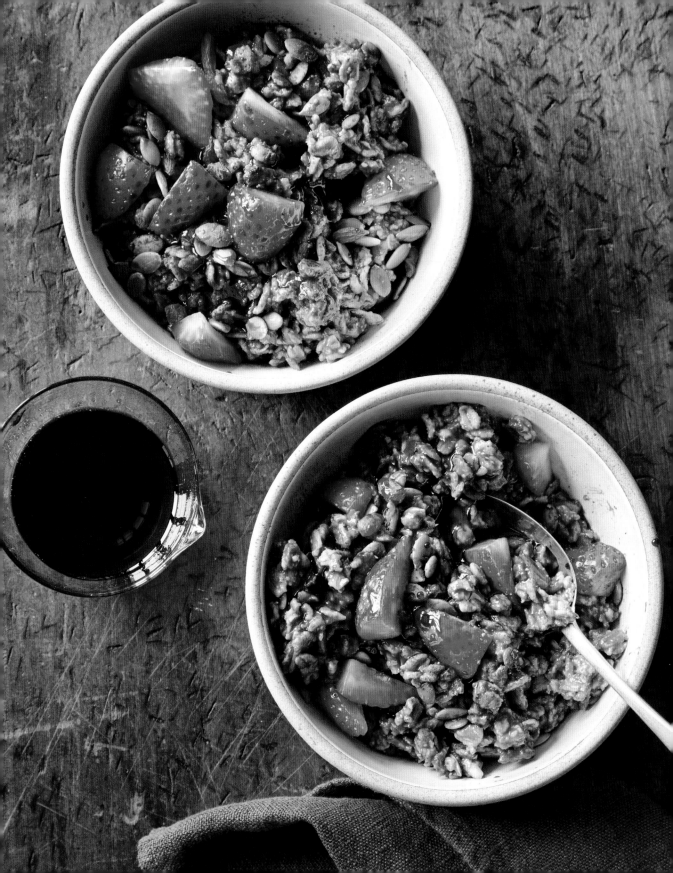

CHOCOLATE OATMEAL

MAKES: *4* (1-CUP) SERVINGS · DIFFICULTY: *easy*

Get creative with this recipe! Mix and match your favorite toppings, such as fresh berries and other fruits, chopped nuts, or swirls of almond butter or peanut butter.

1½ cups old-fashioned rolled oats

3 to 4 tablespoons unsweetened cocoa powder

½ teaspoon ground cinnamon

2 tablespoons chopped dried figs, goji berries, or barberries

1 tablespoon ground flaxseeds

1 tablespoon pumpkin seeds

2 tablespoons raisins (optional)

2 tablespoons Date Syrup (page 3)

In a saucepan, bring 3 cups of water to a boil and then stir in the oats, cocoa powder, and cinnamon. Reduce the heat to low, add the figs, cover, and simmer for 5 minutes, stirring occasionally. Remove from the heat. Stir in the flaxseeds and pumpkin seeds. Cover and let stand for 2 minutes. To serve, spoon the oatmeal into bowls and top with the raisins (if using) and Date Syrup.

Daily Dozen Foods

✗ BERRIES ✗ OTHER FRUITS ✗ FLAXSEEDS ✗ NUTS AND SEEDS ✗ HERBS AND SPICES ✗ WHOLE GRAINS

MORNING GRAIN BOWLS

MAKES: *4* SERVINGS · DIFFICULTY: *easy*

Leftover cooked grains are a great way to start the day—and quick, too! If you don't have leftover grains, cook up a pot of your favorite grain the day before and you'll have the start of something good in the morning.

3 cups cooked whole grains (brown rice, quinoa, freekeh, or oats)

¾ cup cooked cannellini beans, mashed

2 cups Almond Milk (page 2)

3 tablespoons ground flaxseeds

1 1-inch piece fresh turmeric, grated (or 1 teaspoon ground)

1 teaspoon grated fresh ginger (optional)

1 cup fresh or thawed frozen mixed berries

1 ripe banana, peeled and sliced

4 tablespoons Date Syrup (page 3) (optional)

In a microwave-safe bowl, combine the cooked grains, beans, Almond Milk, flaxseeds, turmeric, and ginger (if using). Mix well. Microwave for 2 to 3 minutes, or until warm but not too hot. Divide the grain mixture among four bowls. Top each serving with ¼ cup of the berries and one-quarter of the sliced banana. Drizzle each serving with 1 tablespoon of Date Syrup, if desired.

Daily Dozen Foods

✗ BEANS   ✗ BERRIES   ✗ OTHER FRUITS   ✗ FLAXSEEDS   ✗ HERBS AND SPICES   ✗ WHOLE GRAINS

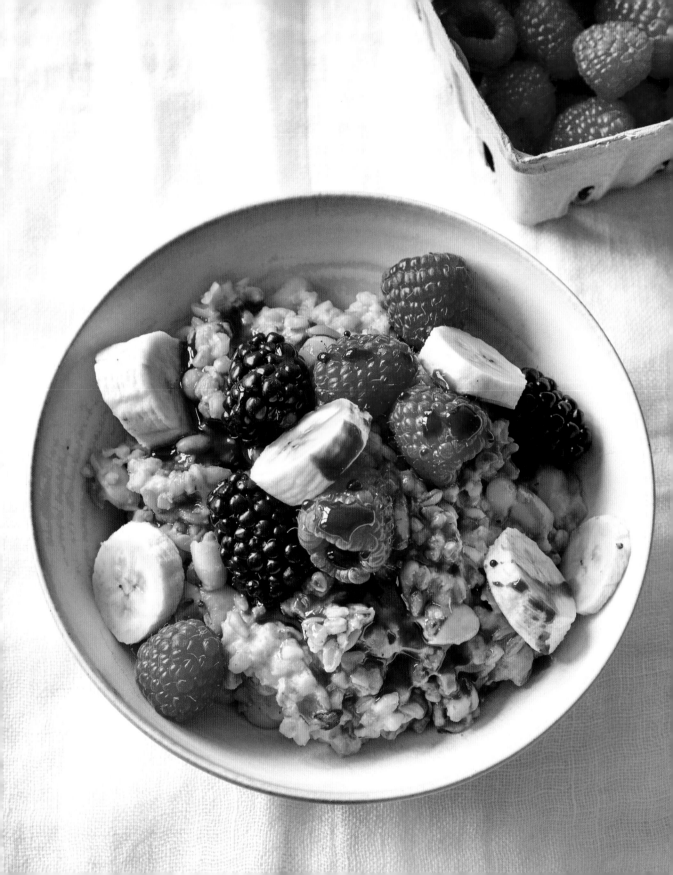

BURRITO BREAKFAST BAKE

MAKES: *4* SERVINGS · DIFFICULTY: *moderate*

Baked sweet potatoes are one of my favorites—whether eaten as-is, spiced and seasoned, or featured in a dish like this one. To save time, I like to bake extras and keep them on hand or, in a pinch, quickly "bake" one in the microwave.

½ cup chopped red onion

1 orange or red bell pepper, finely chopped

6 cups chopped spinach, red chard, or red kale

1 teaspoon Savory Spice Blend (page 4)

1 teaspoon chili powder

½ teaspoon ground cumin

½ teaspoon dried oregano

2 cups Summer Salsa (page 41) or your favorite salt-free salsa

1½ cups cooked or 1 15.5-ounce BPA-free can or Tetra Pak* salt-free black beans, drained and rinsed

1 baked sweet potato, mashed

2 tablespoons minced fresh cilantro

2 tablespoons nutritional yeast

4 salt-free 100% whole-grain tortillas

¼ cup coarsely ground pumpkin seeds

1 ripe Hass avocado, diced (optional)

1 fresh jalapeño pepper, chopped (optional)

Preheat the oven to 350°F.

Combine the onion and bell pepper in a large saucepan with ¼ cup of water over medium heat. Cook for 5 minutes to soften. Add the greens, stirring until wilted and the water is evaporated. Add the Savory Spice Blend, chili powder, cumin, oregano, and ¼ cup of the Summer Salsa, stirring to combine. Remove from the heat.

Mash the black beans in a large bowl. Add the reserved vegetable mixture and stir to mix well.

In a separate bowl, combine the mashed sweet potato, cilantro, nutritional yeast, and ¼ cup of the salsa.

Spoon ¾ cup of the salsa into a 9 × 13-inch baking dish, spreading evenly. Set aside.

Spoon one-quarter of the sweet potato mixture down the center of each tortilla. Top each with one-quarter of the bean mixture. Roll up the tortillas and arrange them, seam side down, in the prepared baking dish. Spread the remaining ¾ cup of salsa over the burritos. Sprinkle with the pumpkin seeds. Cover and bake for 20 to 30 minutes, or until hot. Serve hot, garnished with diced avocado and chopped jalapeño, if desired.

* Tetra Pak is a type of aseptic packaging, meaning free from contamination from bacteria and other microorganisms, so the foods have very long shelf lives.

Daily Dozen Foods

X BEANS   X GREENS   X OTHER VEGETABLES   X NUTS AND SEEDS   X HERBS AND SPICES   X WHOLE GRAINS

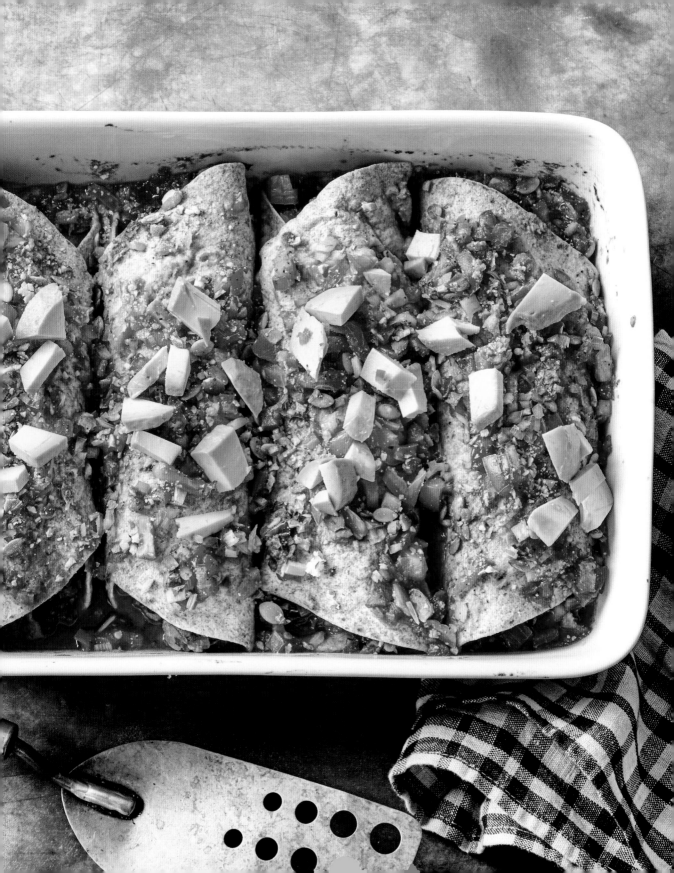

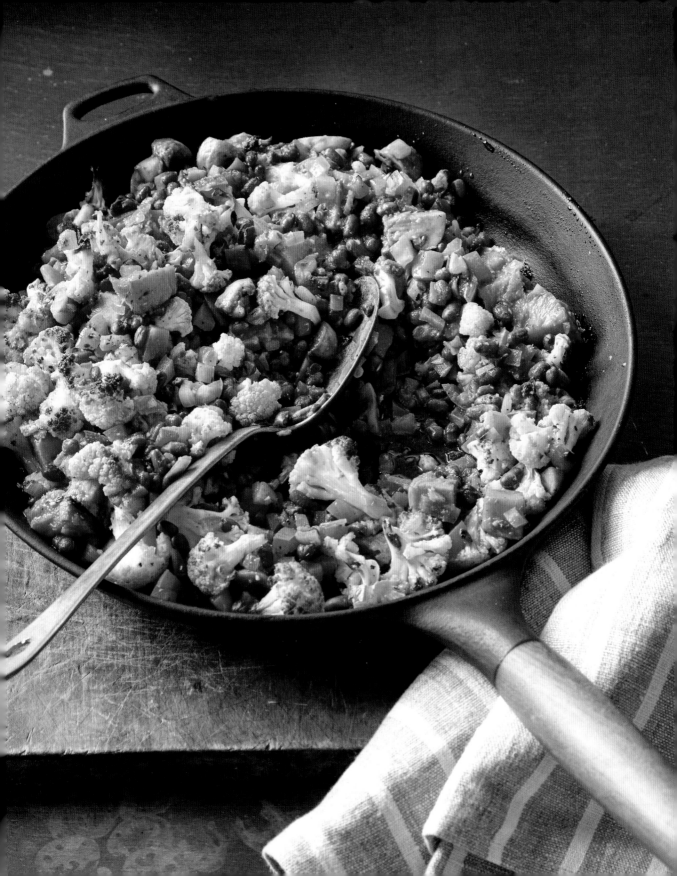

SKILLET SWEET POTATO HASH

MAKES: *4* (1¼-CUP) SERVINGS · DIFFICULTY: *easy*

Although this recipe is in the Breakfast chapter, it's a rousing hit any time of the day or night. Make your Savory Spice Blend and Umami Sauce in advance to really cut down on the time it takes to prepare this dish. Can we talk spice? I love spicy foods, but know some people don't, so feel free to omit the cayenne. On the other hand, if you want even more heat, don't be shy about adding some Healthy Hot Sauce (page 8) when serving.

1 medium sweet potato, peeled and chopped

2 cups chopped cauliflower

1 small red onion, chopped

1 red bell pepper, chopped

8 ounces mushrooms, coarsely chopped

1½ cups cooked or 1 15.5-ounce BPA-free can or Tetra Pak salt-free black or red beans, drained and rinsed

2 to 3 teaspoons Savory Spice Blend (page 4)

¼ teaspoon cayenne pepper or red pepper flakes, or to taste

3 to 4 tablespoons Umami Sauce (page 5)

Preheat the oven to 425°F and line a baking sheet with a silicone mat or parchment paper. Spread the sweet potato on the prepared baking sheet and roast for 10 minutes; then add the cauliflower to the pan. Continue to roast until the sweet potatoes and cauliflower are tender, about 20 minutes. Remove from the oven and set aside.

Heat 2 tablespoons of water in a large skillet over medium heat. Add the onion, cover, and cook until tender, about 5 minutes. Add the bell pepper and mushrooms and cook, uncovered, stirring until tender, about 5 minutes. Add the beans, Savory Spice Blend, cayenne, and roasted vegetables and cook until heated through, about 5 minutes longer. Mash the ingredients lightly with a spatula, if desired. Drizzle with the Umami Sauce and serve hot.

VARIATION: Mix it up with different veggies. Instead of cauliflower, why not try zucchini or another vegetable of your choosing?

Daily Dozen Foods

✗ BEANS   ✗ CRUCIFEROUS VEGETABLES   ✗ OTHER VEGETABLES   ✗ HERBS AND SPICES

ARTICHOKE-SPINACH DIP

LEMONY HUMMUS

THREE-SEED CRACKERS

PUMPKIN SEED DIP

BLACK-EYED PEAS &
ROASTED RED PEPPER DIP

EDAMAME GUACAMOLE

SUMMER SALSA

CHEESY KALE CRISPS

SMOKY ROASTED CHICKPEAS

THREE

SNACKS, DIPS, AND SPREADS

The recipes in this chapter are some of my all-time favorites when I'm feeling a little peckish and want a light lunch or a between-meal snack. When I'm on the road (or in the air), I often take some Cheesy Kale Crisps or Smoky Roasted Chickpeas with me. If you haven't noticed, convenience is almost as important to me as healthy (and flavorful) eating, which is why I really love the dips and spreads in this section. Each one can be enjoyed spread on Three-Seed Crackers or whole-grain bread, or served with raw veggies.

ARTICHOKE-SPINACH DIP

MAKES: *6* (½-CUP) SERVINGS · DIFFICULTY: *easy*

Artichokes are remarkably high in antioxidants. I consider them too much of a pain to cook from scratch, so artichoke hearts are frequently included on my shopping list. They blend well with so many things, including spinach.

---

9 to 10 ounces fresh or thawed frozen spinach, cooked and cooled

1 cup cooked white beans, drained and rinsed

2 tablespoons nutritional yeast

2 tablespoons minced scallion

1 garlic clove, minced

2 teaspoons blended peeled lemon (see page 3)

2 teaspoons white miso paste

¼ teaspoon ground black pepper

Savory Spice Blend (page 4)

1 14-ounce jar artichoke hearts, drained, or 1 10-ounce package frozen artichokes, cooked and cooled

Three-Seed Crackers (page 34), whole-grain crostini or crackers, or raw veggies, to serve

Preheat the oven to 350°F. Squeeze out the excess moisture from the cooled spinach and set aside. In a food processor, combine 2 table-spoons of water and the white beans, nutritional yeast, scallion, garlic, lemon, miso paste, black pepper, and Savory Spice Blend to taste and process until smooth and well blended. For a creamier texture, add a little more water, 1 tablespoon at a time. Add the artichokes and pulse until they are chopped. Add the spinach and pulse to combine. Transfer to a baking dish and bake until warm, 12 to 15 minutes. Spoon onto crackers or crostini, or serve as a dip for raw veggies.

VARIATION: Thin with some Almond Milk (page 2) or Vegetable Broth (page 6) and use as a sauce for pasta.

A CULINARY EXPLORER

Expand your culinary horizons beyond the many ways we already typically enjoy dips and spreads. Why not include one (or more) in a collard wrap? In the mood for pasta? Thin your favorite dip or spread with Almond Milk (page 2) or Vegetable Broth (page 6) and toss with cooked whole-grain pasta. You can even mix a dip or spread with grains and use it as a delicious stuffing for bell peppers and other veggies. The sky's the limit when it comes to thinking of different ways to incorporate these recipes into your menus.

Daily Dozen Foods

✗ BEANS   ✗ GREENS   ✗ OTHER VEGETABLES   ✗ HERBS AND SPICES

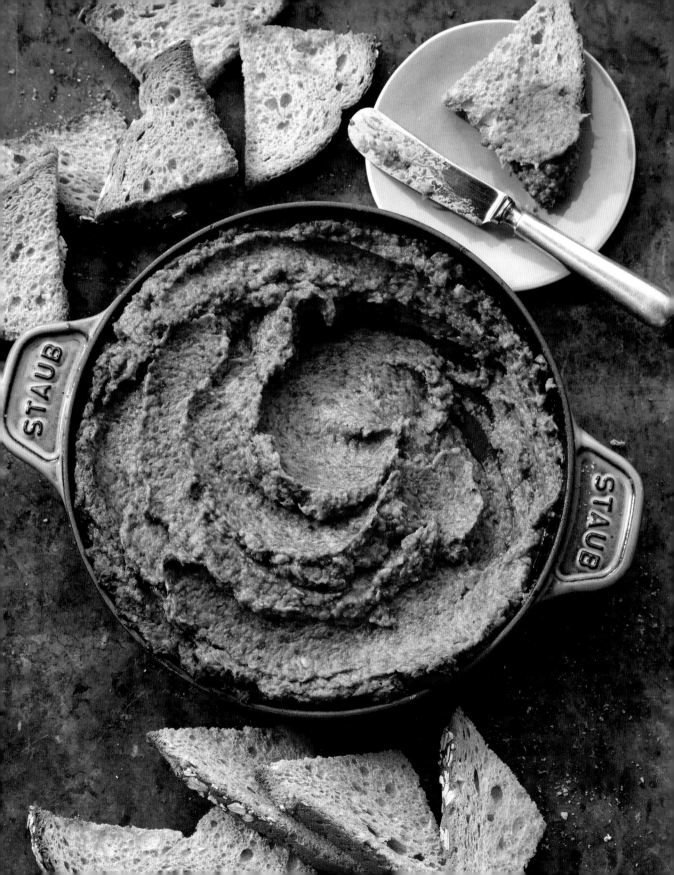

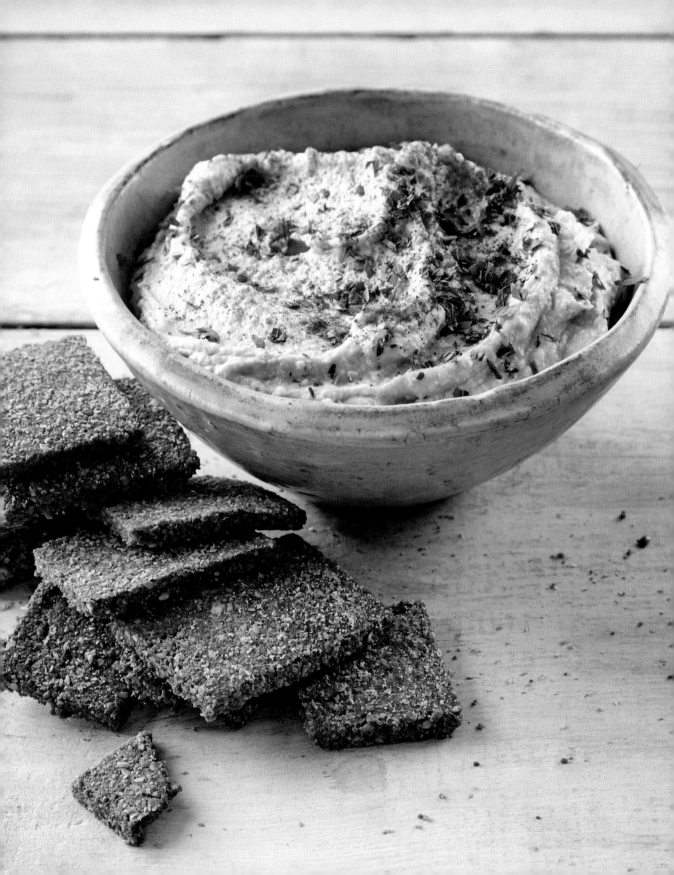

LEMONY HUMMUS

MAKES: ABOUT *2* CUPS · DIFFICULTY: *easy*

It's no secret that hummus is a wonderful dip for raw vegetables and a fantastic spread for collard wraps and other sandwiches . . . but did you know it even tastes great on whole-grain spaghetti? (I admit I've not only put hummus directly on pasta, but I've devoured it!)

2 garlic cloves, crushed

1 tablespoon blended peeled lemon (see page 3)

¼ cup tahini

1 teaspoon white miso paste

1½ cups cooked or 1 15.5-ounce BPA-free can or Tetra Pak salt-free chickpeas, drained and rinsed

¼ teaspoon ground cumin

¼ teaspoon smoked paprika

2 tablespoons chopped fresh parsley

In a food processor, combine the garlic and lemon and process until smooth. Add the tahini and miso paste and process once more until smooth. Add the chickpeas, cumin, and paprika and process for several minutes until very smooth. Add a little water, 1 tablespoon at a time, if a thinner texture is desired. Taste and adjust the seasoning with more lemon or cumin, if needed. To serve, transfer to a bowl and sprinkle with the parsley.

VARIATIONS: Try any or all of these substitutions: replace the chickpeas with black beans or white beans, the parsley with cilantro or dill, and the lemon with lime.

BPA

BPA, which stands for bisphenol A, is an industrial chemical that has been used since the 1950s in various plastic containers and the inside of many metal products, including canned foods. Research has shown that BPA can seep into foods, causing possible negative health effects on the brain and/or heart, and may be linked to diabetes and obesity as well. More research is being undertaken to study BPA, but at the present time there are no federal restrictions on its use in food containers.

What to do? Many companies now make BPA-free containers—these should be clearly labeled. You might also consider using nonplastic or metal containers, such as glass or stainless steel.

Daily Dozen Foods

✗ BEANS　　✗ NUTS AND SEEDS　　✗ HERBS AND SPICES

THREE-SEED CRACKERS

MAKES: ABOUT *25* (2¼-INCH) SQUARE CRACKERS · DIFFICULTY: *moderate*

Making your own crackers is easier (and more fun) than you might think. As a bonus, you can customize them to suit your taste, adding different seasonings as desired.

½ cup raw pumpkin seeds

½ cup raw sunflower seeds

½ cup sesame seeds

1 ¼-inch piece fresh turmeric, grated (or ¼ teaspoon ground)

¼ cup ground flaxseeds

2 tablespoons minced fresh parsley

1 tablespoon nutritional yeast

1½ teaspoons white miso paste

¼ teaspoon onion powder

1 teaspoon dried basil, dill, oregano, or thyme (optional)

Preheat the oven to 250°F. In a blender or food processor, grind the pumpkin seeds, sunflower seeds, ¼ cup of the sesame seeds, and the turmeric into a powder. Add the remaining ingredients, except the remaining sesame seeds, and pulse to combine and mix into a dough. If the dough is too dry, add up to 1 cup of water, 1 tablespoon at a time.

Spread out the dough flat on a baking sheet lined with a silicone mat or parchment paper. Top with another piece of parchment paper and roll out the dough evenly and thinly with a rolling pin or by pressing with your hands. (The rolled-out dough should be approximately a 12 × 10-inch rectangle.) Remove the top layer of parchment paper. Sprinkle with the remaining ¼ cup of sesame seeds and lightly press them into the cracker dough. Use a sharp knife to score the crackers into the size you desire. Bake until lightly browned, about 3 hours. (For a crisper cracker, leave them in the oven with the heat turned off for a while longer.) Once cooled completely, the crackers may be stored at room temperature in a tightly covered container.

10 WAYS TO USE FLAXSEEDS

Whether you buy flaxseeds preground or grind them at home in a spice grinder, coffee grinder, or blender, you can enjoy this nutty superfood in all sorts of ways.

Here are a handful to get you started:

1. Sprinkle into oatmeal.
2. Shake onto salads.
3. Add to smoothies.
4. Use as a binder in burgers (pages 88 and 98) and loaves (page 156).
5. Add to homemade crackers (see above).
6. Use in your homemade energy bites (page 15).
7. Sprinkle on soups.
8. Use as a binder in baked goods.
9. Sprinkle on grain dishes.
10. Use as a thickener in sauces.

Daily Dozen Foods

✗ **FLAXSEEDS**   ✗ **NUTS AND SEEDS**   ✗ **HERBS AND SPICES**

PUMPKIN SEED DIP

MAKES: *3* CUPS · DIFFICULTY: *easy*

Pumpkin seeds! They are delicious, nutritious, and one of the most concentrated sources of zinc. Here's an interesting fact: Men need more zinc than women. Why? Because men lose zinc in every seminal emission. (Semen is filled with zinc.) In fact, men effectively lose about a quarter-cup's worth of pumpkin seeds every time! No matter your gender or (ahem) how much zinc you may want to replenish, enjoy this dip with raw veggies, as a spread for sandwiches, or thin out and use as sauce for pasta.

1¼ cups raw unsalted pumpkin seeds (pepitas)

3 cloves Roasted Garlic (page 6)

1½ cups cooked or 1 15.5-ounce BPA-free can or Tetra Pak salt-free cannellini beans, drained and rinsed

1 teaspoon minced jalapeño pepper, or to taste (optional)

1 tablespoon tahini or almond butter

2 tablespoons blended peeled lemon (see page 3)

1½ teaspoons white miso paste

1 teaspoon Savory Spice Blend (page 4)

½ teaspoon smoked paprika

3 tablespoons minced fresh cilantro (optional)

Assorted cut raw vegetables, for dipping

Preheat the oven to 250°F. Line a baking sheet with a silicone mat or parchment paper. Spread the pumpkin seeds on the prepared baking sheet and toast for 15 to 18 minutes, or until they begin to lightly brown, stirring occasionally so they don't burn. Remove from the oven and set aside to cool.

Once the pumpkin seeds are cool to the touch, transfer them to a food processor and add the Roasted Garlic, beans, jalapeño (if using), tahini, lemon, miso, Savory Spice Blend, paprika, and 3 tablespoons of water. Process until smooth. Transfer to a bowl and sprinkle with cilantro, if desired. Serve with your favorite raw vegetable dippers.

Daily Dozen Foods

✗ BEANS   ✗ OTHER VEGETABLES   ✗ NUTS AND SEEDS   ✗ HERBS AND SPICES

BLACK-EYED PEAS & ROASTED RED PEPPER DIP

MAKES: ABOUT *3* CUPS · DIFFICULTY: *easy*

Black-eyed peas are as marvelously nutritious as all the other legumes. They can be found frozen, canned, or dried at your local supermarket.

2 roasted red bell peppers (see page 9), or 1 9-ounce jar roasted red peppers, drained

1½ cups cooked or 1 15.5-ounce BPA-free can or Tetra Pak salt-free black-eyed peas, drained and rinsed

2 garlic cloves, crushed

1 teaspoon minced jalapeño pepper, or to taste

3 tablespoons tahini

1 tablespoon blended peeled lemon (see page 3)

1 teaspoon Savory Spice Blend (page 4)

1 teaspoon white miso paste

1 teaspoon smoked paprika

Cut raw vegetables, for dipping

In a food processor, combine the roasted red peppers, black-eyed peas, garlic, and jalapeño and pulse to combine. Add the tahini, lemon, Savory Spice Blend, miso, and paprika and process until smooth. Transfer the dip to a bowl and serve with the raw vegetable dippers.

VARIATIONS: Serve with toasted corn tortillas, or use as a spread for sandwiches or collard wraps.

Daily Dozen Foods

X BEANS   X OTHER VEGETABLES   X NUTS AND SEEDS   X HERBS AND SPICES

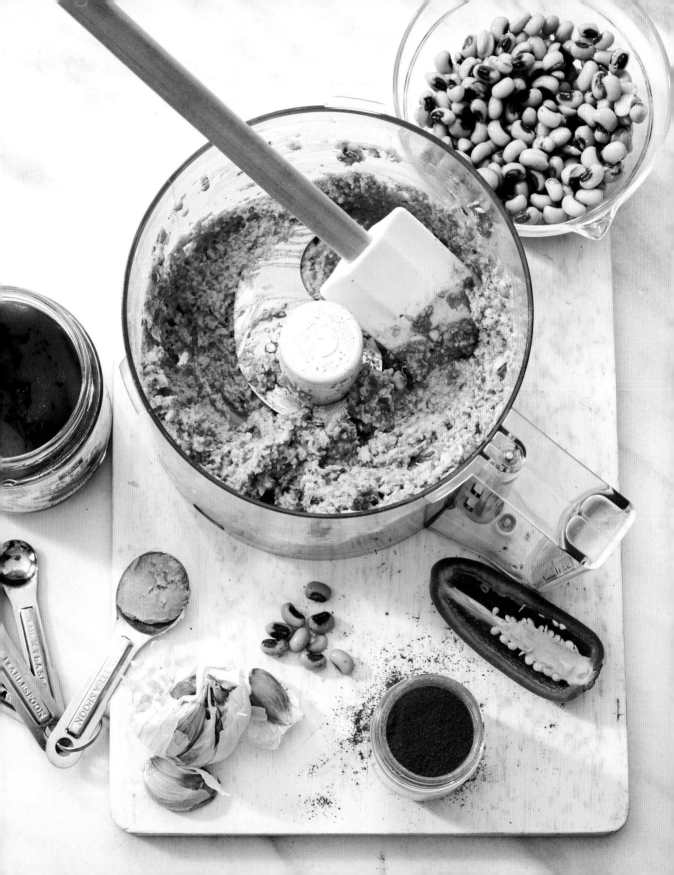

EDAMAME GUACAMOLE

MAKES: ABOUT 1½ CUPS · DIFFICULTY: *easy*

Edamame has been a long-time favorite snack of mine. They're so good I can eat a seemingly endless amount of them right from their pods. This recipe calls for them to be incorporated into a creative take on guacamole, which I love just as much as enjoying them au naturel.

The problem with guacamole is that most people want to dip salted, deep-fried tortilla chips into it. Don't do it! Skip the chip in favor of raw vegetables, such as carrots or bell pepper strips. Or, do as I do, and dip with steamed asparagus.

---

1 cup frozen shelled edamame, thawed

1 ripe Hass avocado, peeled and pitted

2 teaspoons blended peeled lime (see page 3)

1 teaspoon Savory Spice Blend (page 4)

⅛ to ¼ teaspoon ground cumin, or to taste

1 Roma tomato, finely chopped

2 tablespoons chopped fresh cilantro

1 tablespoon minced red onion

1 tablespoon minced jalapeño pepper (optional)

Steamed asparagus or raw vegetables, for dipping

Cook the edamame in a saucepan of boiling water until tender, 10 to 12 minutes. Drain and set aside to cool.

In a food processor, combine the edamame, avocado, lime, Savory Spice Blend, and cumin, and process until smooth. Transfer to a bowl and fold in the tomato, cilantro, onion, and jalapeño (if using). Serve with vegetables for dipping.

Daily Dozen Foods

✗ BEANS   ✗ OTHER FRUITS   ✗ OTHER VEGETABLES   ✗ HERBS AND SPICES

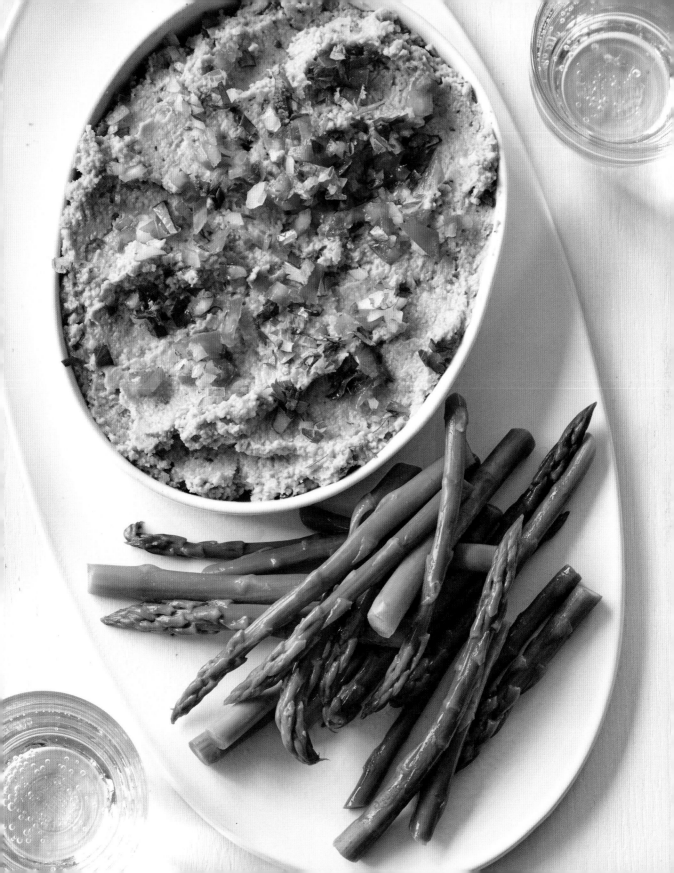

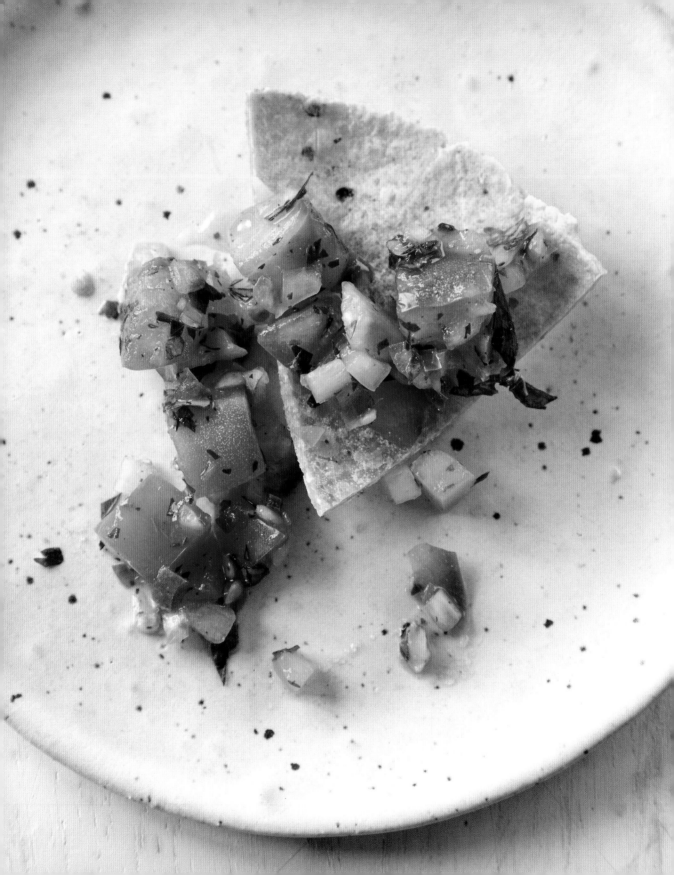

SUMMER SALSA

MAKES: ABOUT *3* CUPS · DIFFICULTY: *easy*

Homemade salsa is best when fresh tomatoes are at their peak. One of my favorite things about making my own salsa is that I can really make it special. Depending on what I'm craving in the moment, I can add as much or as little heat, double or outright skip the cilantro, add such veggies as corn, carrots, and whatever else may tickle my fancy (and my taste buds).

---

6 firm plum tomatoes, cored and coarsely chopped

½ orange or yellow bell pepper, minced

2 tablespoons minced red onion

1 jalapeño or other small hot chili pepper, seeded and minced

2 teaspoons blended peeled lime (see page 3)

2 tablespoons minced fresh cilantro

2 tablespoons minced fresh parsley

Savory Spice Blend (page 4)

In a bowl, combine all the ingredients, adding Savory Spice Blend to taste, and stir well. Cover and let stand at room temperature for 1 hour before serving. If not using right away, store in the refrigerator. The salsa will keep refrigerated for 3 to 4 days.

FRUIT

Although each recipe in this chapter makes a healthy snack, don't forget that nature's best snack food is fruit. Abundant, inexpensive, and healthy, fruit satisfies your midday hunger and tastes great as well. Anyone who thinks it's not convenient to eat plant-based has never met an apple.

Daily Dozen Foods

✗ OTHER VEGETABLES   ✗ HERBS AND SPICES

CHEESY KALE CRISPS

MAKES: *4* (1¼-CUP) SERVINGS · DIFFICULTY: *moderate*

What a great way to eat your greens! Kale, one of the oldest forms of cultivated cabbage, is easy to grow and filled with such dark green leafy goodness. My dear friend Essy (Dr. Caldwell Esselstyn Jr.) eats as much of it and other dark green leafies as he can throughout the day. You'll be seeing kale in many of the recipes in this book—for good reason!

1 bunch red kale, thick stems removed

½ cup raw cashews, soaked for 3 hours and then drained

½ cup roasted red bell pepper (see page 9), or store-bought

3 tablespoons nutritional yeast

1 teaspoon rice vinegar

1 teaspoon white miso paste

1 ¼-inch piece fresh turmeric, grated (or ¼ teaspoon ground)

1 teaspoon smoked paprika

Wash the kale leaves well and then tear or cut any large leaves into 2-inch pieces. Dry the kale pieces in a salad spinner or a clean dish towel. Once the kale is very dry, transfer it to a large bowl and set aside. Preheat the oven to 350°F. Line two large baking sheets with silicone mats and set aside.

In a food processor or high-speed blender, combine 2 tablespoons of water and the remaining ingredients and process until smooth. The sauce should be thick enough to coat the kale. If it's too thick, add a little more water, 1 tablespoon at a time. Pour the sauce onto the kale and toss to coat, massaging the sauce into the leaves. Arrange the kale in a single layer on the prepared baking sheets and bake for 20 minutes. Remove any pieces that are crisp and turn over any that have not yet crisped before returning the trays to the oven for 2 to 5 minutes longer, or until the remaining kale pieces are crisp. Be sure to watch so they don't burn. Set aside to cool completely before eating.

Daily Dozen Foods

✗ GREENS   ✗ OTHER VEGETABLES   ✗ NUTS AND SEEDS   ✗ HERBS AND SPICES

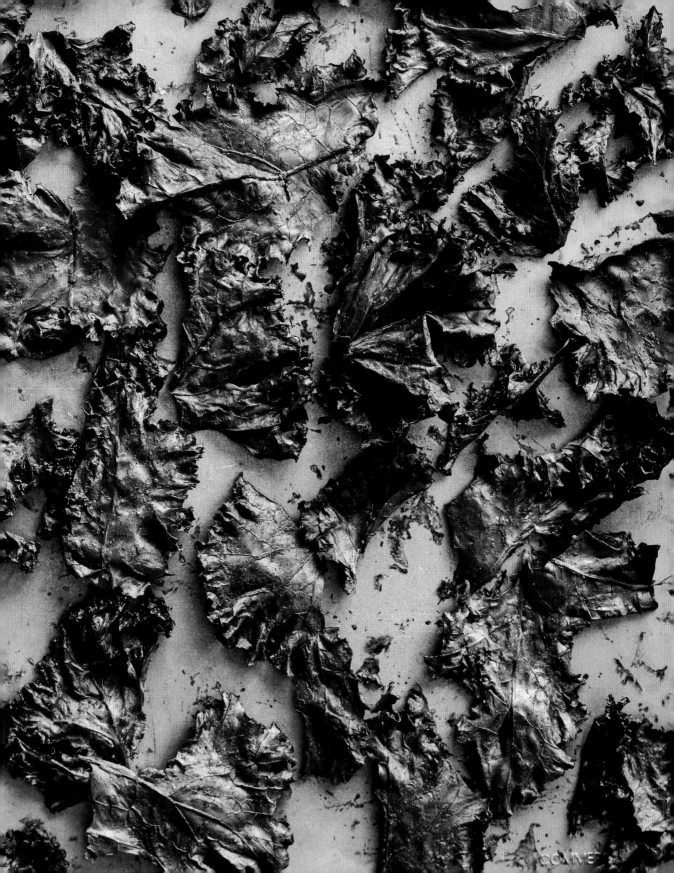

SMOKY ROASTED CHICKPEAS

MAKES ABOUT *1½* CUPS · DIFFICULTY: *easy*

More chickpeas! There are just so many things you can do with these little protein- and fiber-packed legumes. I can't get enough of them, and neither should you!

1½ cups cooked or 1 15.5-ounce BPA-free can or Tetra Pak salt-free chickpeas, drained, well rinsed, and blotted dry

1 tablespoon Date Syrup (page 3)

1 tablespoon nutritional yeast

2 teaspoons white miso paste

1½ teaspoons smoked paprika

¼ teaspoon onion powder

½ teaspoon Savory Spice Blend (page 4)

Preheat the oven to 375°F. Line a baking sheet with a silicone mat or parchment paper and set aside. Make sure the chickpeas are as dry as possible and remove any loose skins.

In a medium bowl, combine 2 tablespoons of water and all the remaining ingredients, except the chickpeas and Savory Spice Blend. Add the chickpeas and toss to coat evenly.

Transfer the chickpeas to the prepared baking sheet, spreading evenly in a single layer. Bake for 30 to 35 minutes, stirring every 8 to 10 minutes, until lightly browned and crunchy. Sprinkle the roasted chickpeas with the spice blend and serve warm or at room temperature. These are best eaten on the day they are made.

POPCORN

One of my all-time favorite snacks is air-popped popcorn with nutritional yeast. If you aren't already familiar it, nutritional yeast is a deactivated yeast (meaning it doesn't grow like baking yeast) and has a cheesy, nutty flavor (as opposed to brewer's yeast, a beer industry by-product that tastes nasty). I just wish it had a better name. Where was the person who came up with "aquafaba" when nutritional yeast was being named? In New Zealand, it's called Brufax. I don't know if that's worse. Those in the know call it "nooch." Okay, that's pretty cute.

Daily Dozen Foods

X BEANS   X HERBS AND SPICES

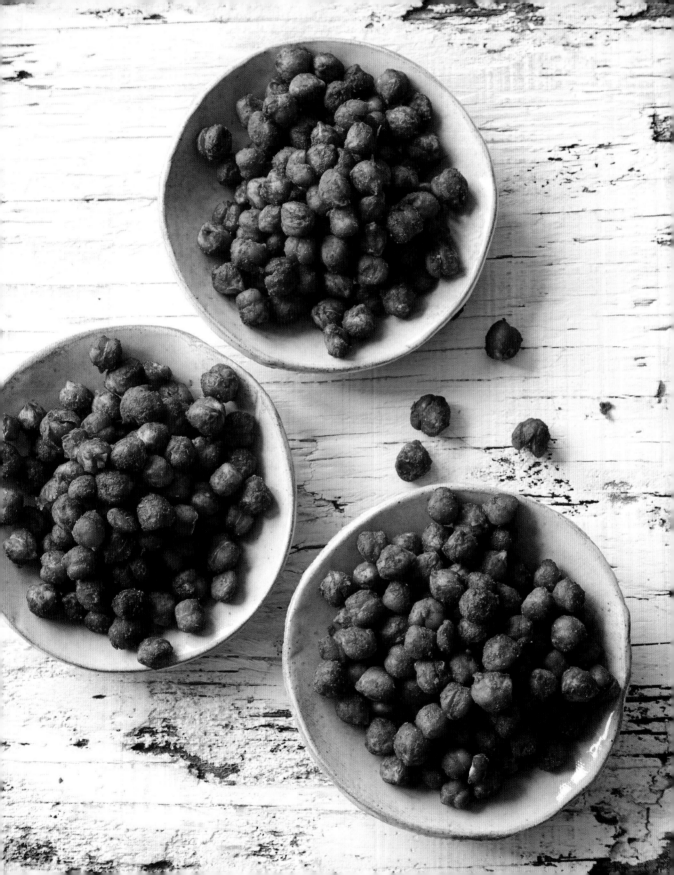

FOUR

SOUPS AND CHILIES

Soups and chilies are the ultimate comfort food. Warming and satisfying, they are a wonderful way to incorporate so many delicious ingredients into a single dish. Start with the hearty bean and vegetable soups and expand your repertoire to Asian-inspired soups and savory chilies.

KALE & WHITE BEAN SOUP

MISO SOUP WITH SPINACH & DULSE

SPICY ASIAN VEGETABLE SOUP

VEGETABLE & RED BEAN GUMBO

BLACK BEAN SOUP WITH QUINOA & KALE

CURRIED CAULIFLOWER SOUP

SUMMER GARDEN GAZPACHO

MOROCCAN LENTIL SOUP

THREE-BEAN CHILI

CHAMPION VEGETABLE CHILI

KALE & WHITE BEAN SOUP

MAKES: *4* (1½-CUP) SERVINGS · DIFFICULTY: *easy*

Kale, kale, and more kale! I can't seem to get enough of it, but if you'd like, feel free to substitute a different variety of greens in this recipe. I think Swiss chard would be delicious!

6 cups Vegetable Broth (page 6)

1 large red onion, chopped

3 to 4 garlic cloves, minced

1 medium sweet potato, cut into ½-inch dice

5 cups chopped fresh red kale

¼ teaspoon red pepper flakes (or more . . . much, much more, if you love spice as I do)

2 bay leaves

1½ cups cooked or 1 15.5-ounce BPA-free can or Tetra Pak salt-free cannellini beans, drained and rinsed

1 teaspoon white miso paste

2 tablespoons nutritional yeast

2 tablespoons chopped fresh parsley

1 teaspoon fresh marjoram or oregano, or ½ teaspoon dried

2 teaspoons Savory Spice Blend (page 4), or to taste

Heat 1 cup of the broth in a large pot over medium heat. Add the onion and garlic and simmer for 5 minutes. Stir in the sweet potato, kale, red pepper flakes, bay leaves, and the remaining 5 cups of broth and bring to a boil over high heat. Lower the heat to medium, add the beans, and cook until the vegetables are tender, 20 to 30 minutes. Ladle about ⅓ cup of the broth into a small bowl or cup. Add the miso paste and stir to blend. Pour the miso mixture into the soup and stir in the nutritional yeast, parsley, marjoram, and Savory Spice Blend. Serve hot.

Daily Dozen Foods

X BEANS   X GREENS   X OTHER VEGETABLES   X HERBS AND SPICES

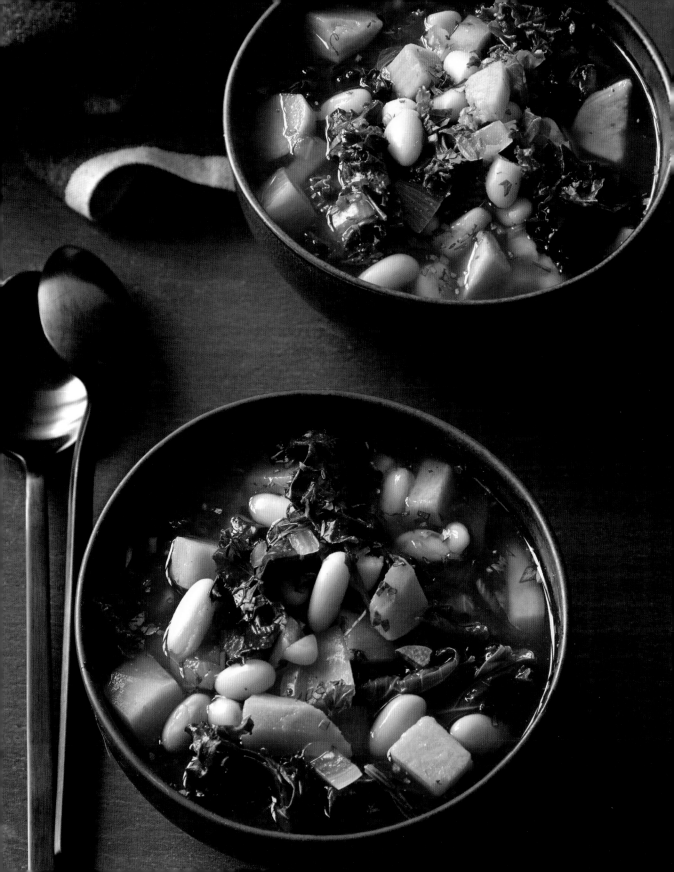

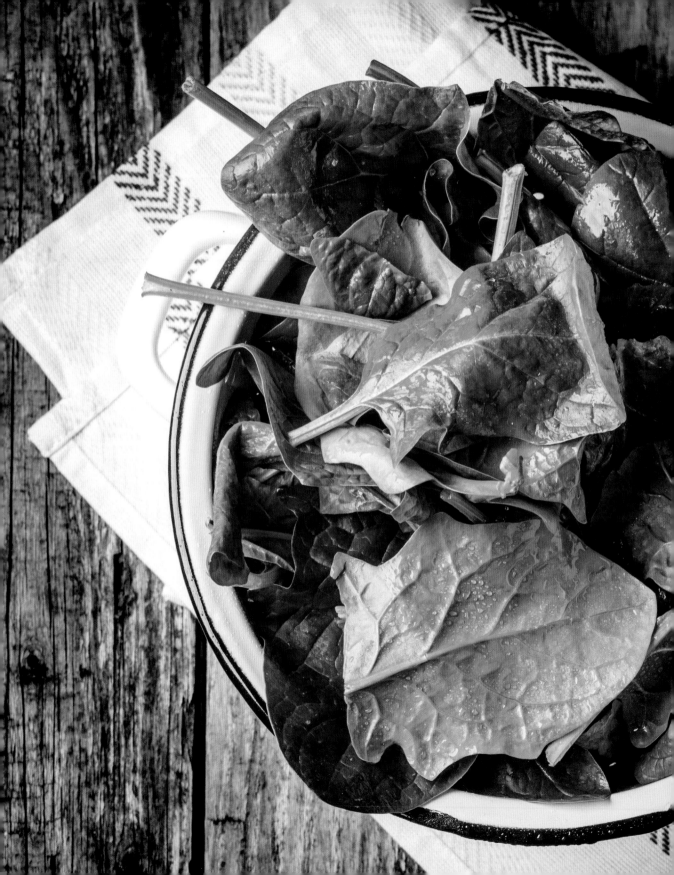

MISO SOUP WITH SPINACH & DULSE

MAKES: *4* SERVINGS • DIFFICULTY: *easy*

One of the milder tasting seaweeds, dried dulse is a good gateway plant to the world of sea vegetables, underwater dark green leafies. Seaweeds aren't just flavorful; they're rich with nutrients, including iodine, which is especially critical for pregnant women. I used to get regular doses of iodine from the Eden brand beans I favored, as the company cans its beans with a bit of seaweed called kombu. Since I started pressure-cooking my own beans, I've gotten into the habit of snacking on sheets of seaweed called nori. You can find nori in a variety of flavors with all sorts of seasonings. I used to play around and season my own, but I've taken to simply eating them straight. Two sheets a day should be all the iodine you need.

3 tablespoons dried dulse, soaked in water for 3 minutes, then drained

5 cups Vegetable Broth (page 6)

1 cup shelled edamame, fresh or thawed if frozen

6 shiitake mushroom caps, thinly sliced

3 scallions, chopped

¼ cup white miso paste

4 cups fresh spinach, cut into strips

Savory Spice Blend (page 4)

Chop the dulse and set aside. Heat the broth in a large saucepan over high heat and bring to a boil. Add the edamame and lower the heat to medium. Simmer for 5 minutes, stir in the mushrooms and scallions, and simmer for 5 minutes longer. Reduce the heat to low. In a small bowl, mix together the miso paste with about ⅓ cup of the hot broth, blending well. Add the blended miso mixture to the soup. Add the dulse, spinach, and Savory Spice Blend to taste and simmer for about 3 minutes. Do not boil. Serve hot.

Daily Dozen Foods

X BEANS   X GREENS   X OTHER VEGETABLES   X HERBS AND SPICES

SPICY ASIAN VEGETABLE SOUP

MAKES: *4* (1¾-CUP) SERVINGS · DIFFICULTY: *easy*

For an even heartier version of this amazing soup, add cooked 100% buckwheat noodles or brown, black, or red rice just before serving.

---

5 cups Vegetable Broth (page 6)

1 4-inch piece lemongrass, crushed

4 tablespoons grated fresh ginger

1 garlic clove, minced

2 cups sliced shiitake mushroom caps

2 shallots, cut lengthwise into thin slivers

2 cups thinly sliced bok choy or napa cabbage

1 cup shredded carrot

3 scallions, chopped

2 teaspoons blended peeled lime (see page 3), or to taste

4 cherry or grape tomatoes, halved

1 teaspoon Healthy Hot Sauce (page 8), or to taste

2 teaspoons Savory Spice Blend (page 4), or to taste

2 tablespoons chopped fresh Thai basil or cilantro

In a large pot, combine the broth, lemongrass, ginger, and garlic. Bring to a boil, then reduce the heat to low, cover, and simmer for 20 minutes. Remove the lemongrass and bring to a boil. Add the mushrooms, shallots, bok choy, and carrot. Reduce the heat to low and cook for 3 minutes. Stir in the scallions, lime, tomatoes, Healthy Hot Sauce, and Savory Spice Blend. Simmer until hot, about 2 minutes. Garnish with Thai basil or cilantro and serve hot.

Daily Dozen Foods

✗ CRUCIFEROUS VEGETABLES   ✗ OTHER VEGETABLES   ✗ HERBS AND SPICES

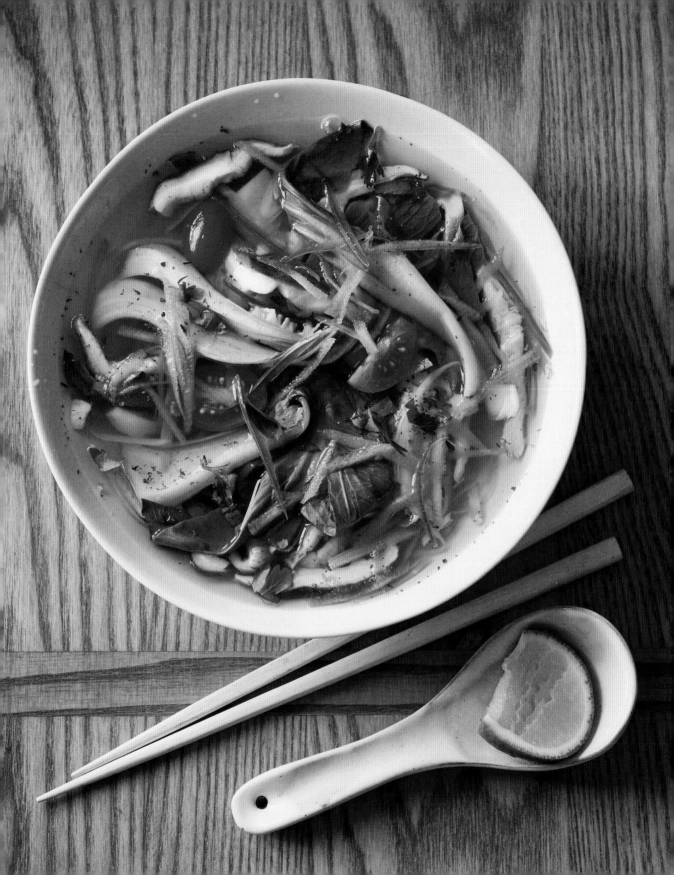

VEGETABLE & RED BEAN GUMBO

MAKES: *4* (1¼-CUP) SERVINGS · DIFFICULTY: *easy*

Some people swear by okra, and others are more than happy to do without it. If you're not okra's biggest fan, skip it and just add more zucchini or green beans to this rich stew. But okra is packed with cholesterol-lowering soluble fiber, so I encourage you to give it one more try before you give it a hard pass.

6 cups Vegetable Broth (page 6) or water

1 medium red onion, chopped

1 green bell pepper, seeded and chopped

½ cup celery, minced

2 or 3 garlic cloves, minced

1 14.5-ounce BPA-free can or Tetra Pak salt-free diced tomatoes, undrained

1½ cups sliced okra, fresh or thawed if frozen

1 cup diced zucchini or cut green beans

3 teaspoons fresh thyme, or 1 teaspoon dried

1 teaspoon dried marjoram or oregano, or 3 teaspoons fresh

1 teaspoon smoked paprika

2 teaspoons salt-free Cajun seasoning (optional)

1½ cups cooked or 1 15.5-ounce BPA-free can or Tetra Pak salt-free dark red kidney beans or black-eyed peas, drained and rinsed

½ teaspoon red pepper flakes, or to taste

2 teaspoons Savory Spice Blend (page 4), or to taste

3 cups cooked brown, black, or red rice, to serve (see note)

Heat 1 cup of the broth in a large pot over medium-high heat. Add the onion, bell pepper, celery, and garlic and cook for 5 minutes, stirring occasionally. Stir in the tomatoes with their juices, okra, zucchini, thyme, marjoram, paprika, and Cajun seasoning (if using). Add the remaining 5 cups of broth and bring to a boil. Lower the heat to a simmer, stir in the beans, and cook until the vegetables are tender, 20 to 30 minutes. Stir in the red pepper flakes and Savory Spice Blend. Serve hot in shallow bowls over the cooked rice.

NOTE: Due to recent studies on the arsenic content in rice, Dr. Greger now recommends diversifying your grains. Wherever a recipe calls for rice, please consider using other whole intake grains, such as quinoa, millet, oat groats, hulled (not pearled) barley, buckwheat, or wheat berries.

Daily Dozen Foods

✗ BEANS   ✗ OTHER VEGETABLES   ✗ HERBS AND SPICES   ✗ WHOLE GRAINS

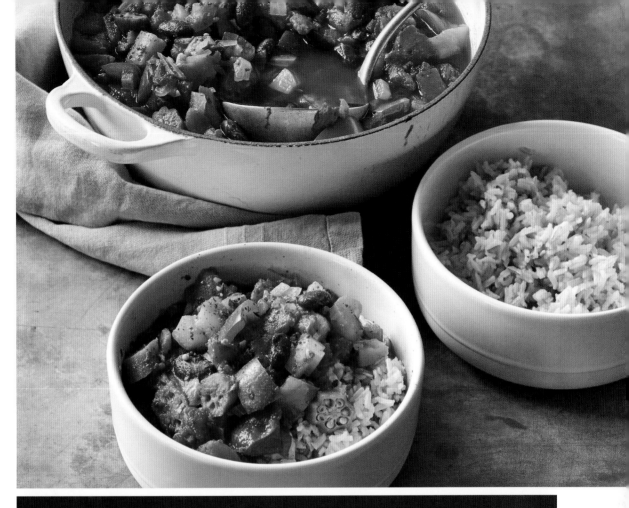

SO MANY PLANTS...

To give you a sense of the variety of healthy foods out there, let me tell you a funny story about the love of my life, Andrea. (Bet you thought I was going to say kale!) When we were first dating ages ago and friends would ask me what she was like, I'd share this with them, as I felt it best summed up her joie de vivre: Andrea decided early on that life was too short to eat the same meal twice. And I mean, *ever*. This was just part of her perpetual seize-the-day attitude, and it

continues today. Every week, she pulls out cookbooks and charts out new recipes for each main meal, making sure to pencil in a notation at the bottom of each so she doesn't forget and accidently make the same dish some years in the future. The most endearing part is that she thinks everyone else is weird for not sharing her passion for culinary adventure.

Of course, cooking for her became a challenge. Whenever I made something I really liked, it came with a degree of

sadness, because I knew we'd never be able to have that dish again. (Although one time I was able to sneak in a repeat performance of my tried-and-true Green Light Mac & Cheese (page 143) by disguising it with enough blended spinach to turn it bright green, and she was none the wiser. Shhh!) The good news is there are so many wonderful whole-plant foods that Andrea can maintain her never-repeat-a-meal habit for the rest of her long, long life.

BLACK BEAN SOUP WITH QUINOA & KALE

MAKES: *4* (2-CUP) SERVINGS • DIFFICULTY: *easy*

Quinoa is a relatively new addition to my diet. I had been looking for different whole grains I could add to my pantry and discovered this gem. When you're at the market, look for the colored varieties, such as red or black quinoa. In fact, I always look for color to get the added benefit of the antioxidant power of the plant pigments. So, I buy red or black rice rather than brown (and never white) and always pick red onions over white and purple cabbage over green.

---

4 cups Vegetable Broth (page 6)

1 red onion, chopped

1 carrot, chopped

1 celery rib, chopped

2 garlic cloves, minced

1 sweet potato, peeled and chopped

1 bay leaf

⅓ cup quinoa, rinsed and drained

3 cups cooked black beans or 2 15.5-ounce BPA-free cans or Tetra Paks black beans, drained and rinsed

1 14.5-ounce BPA-free can or Tetra Pak diced, unsalted tomatoes, undrained

2 teaspoons Savory Spice Blend (page 4)

1 teaspoon ground cumin

½ teaspoon dried oregano

Ground black pepper, to taste

3 cups chopped red kale

In a large pot, heat 1 cup of the broth over medium-high heat. Add the onion, carrot, celery, garlic, and sweet potato. Cook, stirring occasionally, until the vegetables have softened, about 5 minutes. Add the bay leaf, quinoa, beans, tomatoes, Savory Spice Blend, herbs, black pepper, and the remaining 3 cups of broth and bring to a boil. Lower the heat to a simmer and stir in the kale. Cover and cook until the quinoa and vegetables are tender, about 30 minutes. Remove and discard the bay leaf, and serve hot.

KALE

Researchers have found that kale may help control cholesterol levels. In one study, kale substantially lowered participants' bad (LDL) cholesterol and boosted their good (HDL) cholesterol[107] as much as running 300 miles.[108] Although it has been recently called into question whether raising HDL cholesterol actually makes a difference,[109] I still think kale is the bee's knees and well worthy of its nickname "queen of greens."

Daily Dozen Foods

X BEANS X GREENS X OTHER VEGETABLES X HERBS AND SPICES X WHOLE GRAINS

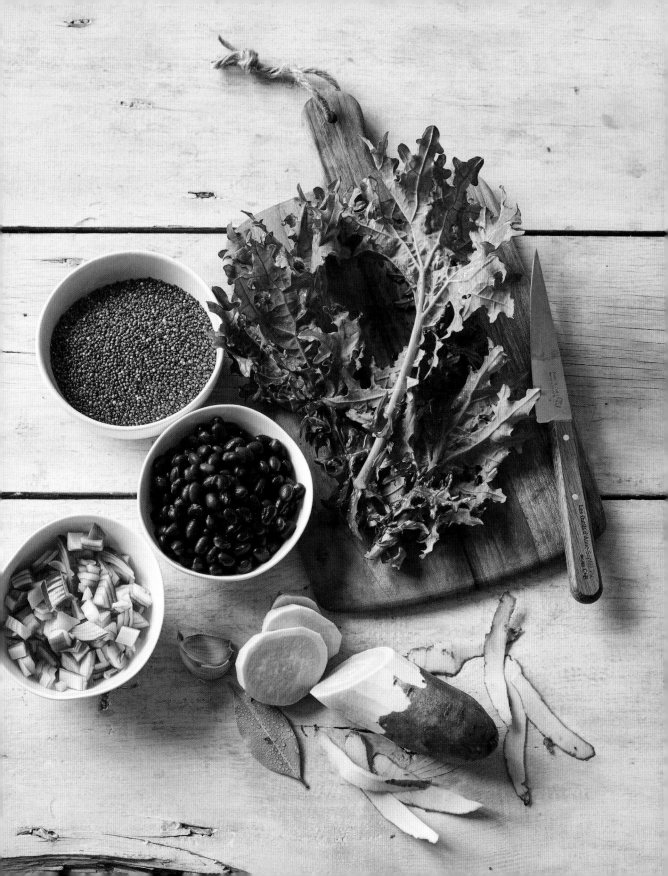

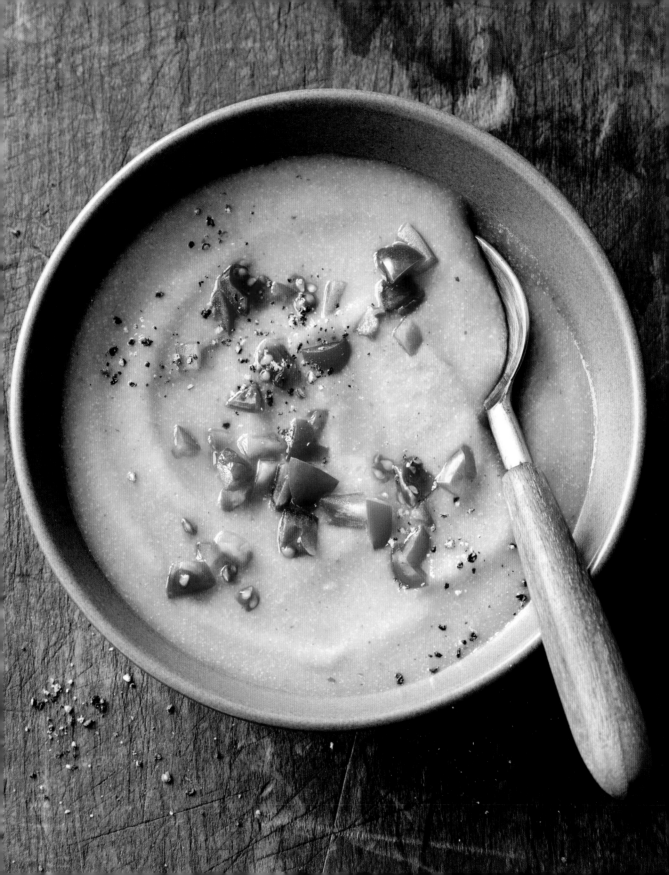

CURRIED CAULIFLOWER SOUP

MAKES: *4* (1¾-CUP) SERVINGS · DIFFICULTY: *easy*

Cauliflower is one of two great exceptions to the white foods rule. Yes, I opt for color to take advantage of the antioxidant boost from plant pigments and shun refined grains, such as white bread and white rice, but although cauliflower might be white, just like its cruciferous cousins, it's one of the healthiest vegetables. (The other unusually healthy white food? White mushrooms.)

4 cups Vegetable Broth (page 6)

1 red onion, chopped

1 garlic clove, minced

1½ teaspoons grated fresh ginger

1½ tablespoons curry powder

2 teaspoons date sugar

1 teaspoon Savory Spice Blend (page 4)

1 head cauliflower, trimmed and coarsely chopped

2 teaspoons blended peeled lemon (see page 3)

1 plum tomato, finely chopped, for garnish

In a large pot, heat 1 cup of the broth over medium-high heat. Add the onion and cook until softened, about 5 minutes. Stir in the garlic, ginger, curry, date sugar, and Savory Spice Blend. Add the cauliflower and the remaining 3 cups of broth and bring to a boil. Lower the heat to a simmer, cover, and cook until the cauliflower is soft, about 30 minutes.

Purée the soup in a food processor or blender, working in batches if necessary, or use a stick blender to purée the soup directly in the pot. Stir in the lemon; then taste and adjust the seasonings as desired. Ladle into bowls and serve hot, garnished with chopped tomato.

VARIATIONS: When ready to serve, add any of the following for a slightly different take on what will surely become a favorite: cooked brown, red, or black rice; green peas; chopped cooked spinach; minced chives; or diced scallion.

Daily Dozen Foods

X CRUCIFEROUS VEGETABLES   X OTHER VEGETABLES   X HERBS AND SPICES

SUMMER GARDEN GAZPACHO

MAKES: *4* SERVINGS · DIFFICULTY: *easy*

By adding cannellini beans to this refreshing gazpacho, you'll create a more satisfying soup.

2 large tomatoes, halved and cored

1 small red bell pepper, halved and seeded

¼ cup coarsely chopped sweet red onion

1 cup chopped cucumber

1 small yellow bell pepper, seeded and chopped

1 garlic clove, minced

1 chili pepper, seeded and minced (and as spicy as you can handle)

2 tablespoons minced scallion

3 tablespoons rice vinegar

1 teaspoon Healthy Hot Sauce (page 8) (optional)

2½ cups unsalted vegetable juice blend, such as V-12 Vegetable Blast (page 219)

¼ cup minced fresh parsley

1 ¼-inch piece fresh turmeric, grated (or ¼ teaspoon ground)

Savory Spice Blend (page 4)

1½ cups cooked or 1 15.5-ounce BPA-free can or Tetra Pak salt-free cannellini beans, drained and rinsed (optional)

1 teaspoon blended peeled lemon (see page 3)

In a blender or food processor, combine the tomatoes, red bell pepper, and onion and process until smooth. Pour the vegetable mixture into a large bowl and stir in the cucumber, yellow bell pepper, garlic, chili, and scallion. Add the vinegar and Healthy Hot Sauce (if using), and stir in the vegetable juice blend, 2 tablespoons of the parsley, the turmeric, and Savory Spice Blend to taste. Stir in the beans (if using). Cover the bowl and refrigerate at least 2 hours to chill and allow flavors to develop. Just before serving, stir in the lemon to brighten the flavors. Serve the soup chilled and garnished with the remaining parsley.

Daily Dozen Foods

✗ BEANS (OPTIONALLY)   ✗ OTHER VEGETABLES   ✗ HERBS AND SPICES

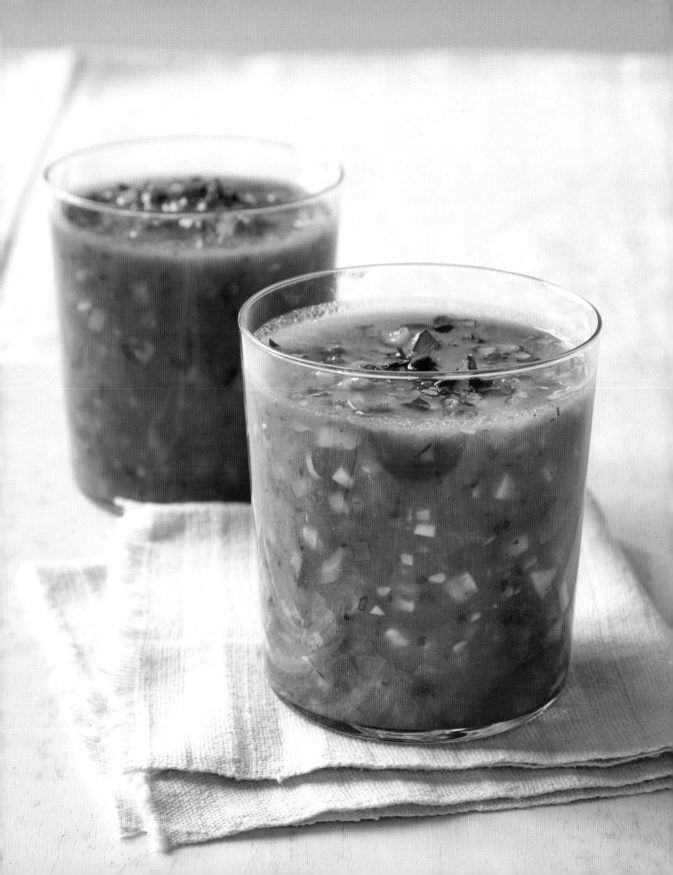

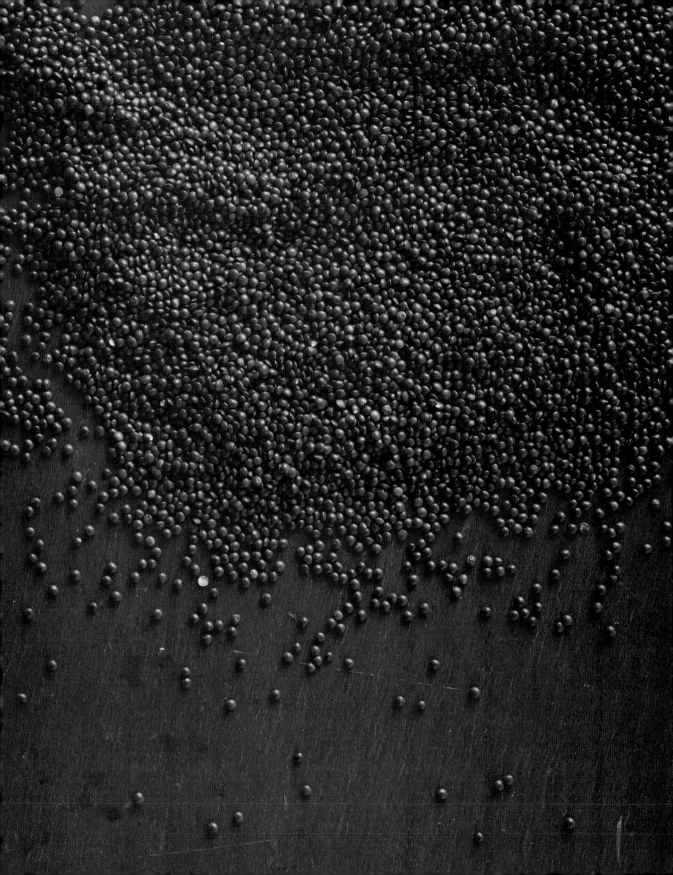

MOROCCAN LENTIL SOUP

MAKES: *4* (1¼-CUP) SERVINGS · DIFFICULTY: *easy*

Lentils are my favorite legume. They cook so quickly, mix well with just about everything, and are exceptionally nutrient dense. I never prepare rice or other grains without throwing in some lentils. Don't forget that any dish can be made healthier by adding beans or greens. A variety of herbs and spices elevate this particular lentil soup from simple to sensational.

5 cups Vegetable Broth (page 6) or water

1 red onion, chopped

2 garlic cloves, chopped

1 red bell pepper, chopped

1 teaspoon grated fresh ginger

1 teaspoon ground coriander

½ teaspoon ground cumin

½ teaspoon ground cinnamon

1 (¼-inch) piece fresh turmeric, grated, or ¼ teaspoon ground turmeric

¼ teaspoon red pepper flakes

¼ teaspoon ground fennel seeds

1 cup dried black or red lentils

1 14.5-ounce BPA-free can or Tetra Pak salt-free diced tomatoes, undrained

1 teaspoon Savory Spice Blend (page 4), or to taste

4 cups chopped baby greens

In a large pot, heat 1 cup of the broth over medium heat. Add the onion, garlic, and bell pepper. Cook until slightly softened, about 5 minutes. Add the ginger, coriander, cumin, cinnamon, turmeric, red pepper flakes, and fennel seeds; then stir in the lentils, tomatoes, and remaining 4 cups of broth. Bring to a boil. Lower the heat to a simmer, cover, and cook until the lentils are soft, 15 to 20 minutes. Add the Savory Spice Blend and stir in the baby greens, simmering until wilted. Serve hot.

COOKING WITH SPICE

With all the exotic, exciting, and excellent spices at the market, you have no excuse not to go out and experiment with new flavors. Myself, I have become very fond of smoked paprika. It's not as easy to find as regular paprika, so I order it online. As much as I love greens, greens with smoked paprika are even better. I'm also very fond of Ceylon cinnamon. I take packets of unsweetened cocoa powder and cinnamon whenever I travel, to make bad hotel coffee taste better. I am also a fan of black pepper. Not the most mysterious of spices, it's a favored staple for a reason. It's so good!

Cooking with spices means paying attention, though. I once made what became known in my family as cardamom death muffins. I was following a recipe for blueberry muffins that called for a bit of dried cardamom. As I prepared my batter, I used the right amount of cardamom, but fresh, not dried. Oh, *wow*, was that a mistake! The muffins were so overpowering that after just one bite, our eyes started watering. I would have figured the dried spice, being concentrated, would be more potent than fresh. Not so!

Daily Dozen Foods

✗ BEANS   ✗ GREENS   ✗ OTHER VEGETABLES   ✗ HERBS AND SPICES

THREE-BEAN CHILI

MAKES: *4* (1¼-CUP) SERVINGS · DIFFICULTY: *easy*

Enjoy this tasty chili alone or on a bed of brown, red, or black rice or cooked greens (or both). It's also a great topping for sweet potatoes.

2 cups Vegetable Broth (page 6)

1 red onion, chopped

1 bell pepper (any color), seeded and chopped

2 garlic cloves, minced

1 small hot chili pepper, seeded and minced

2 to 3 cups chopped mushrooms

2 tablespoons chili powder, or to taste

¼ cup jarred tomato paste

1 14.5-ounce BPA-free can or Tetra Pak salt-free diced tomatoes, undrained

½ cup dried red lentils

1½ cups cooked or 1 15.5-ounce BPA-free can or Tetra Pak salt-free kidney beans, drained and rinsed

1½ cups cooked or 1 15.5-ounce BPA-free can or Tetra Pak salt-free black beans, drained and rinsed

2 tablespoons Umami Sauce (page 5)

1 ¼-inch piece fresh turmeric, grated (or ¼ teaspoon ground)

1 tablespoon Savory Spice Blend (page 4), or to taste

½ teaspoon smoked paprika

¼ teaspoon ground black pepper

In a large pot, heat 1 cup of the broth over medium heat. Add the onion and bell pepper and cook until softened, stirring occasionally, about 5 minutes. Add the garlic, minced chili, and mushrooms; then stir in the chili powder and tomato paste. Add the remaining ingredients, including the second cup of broth, and simmer, stirring occasionally, until the lentils are tender and the flavors are blended, about 50 minutes. Taste to adjust the seasonings, if needed, and serve hot.

CHILI VARIATIONS

Just as there are countless ways to make chili, there are just as many ways to serve it. Try it on a bed of cooked greens or whole grains. Use it as a taco filling. Toss it with whole wheat pasta. Top baked sweet potatoes or winter squash with it. Experiment and enjoy!

Daily Dozen Foods

X BEANS   X OTHER VEGETABLES   X HERBS AND SPICES

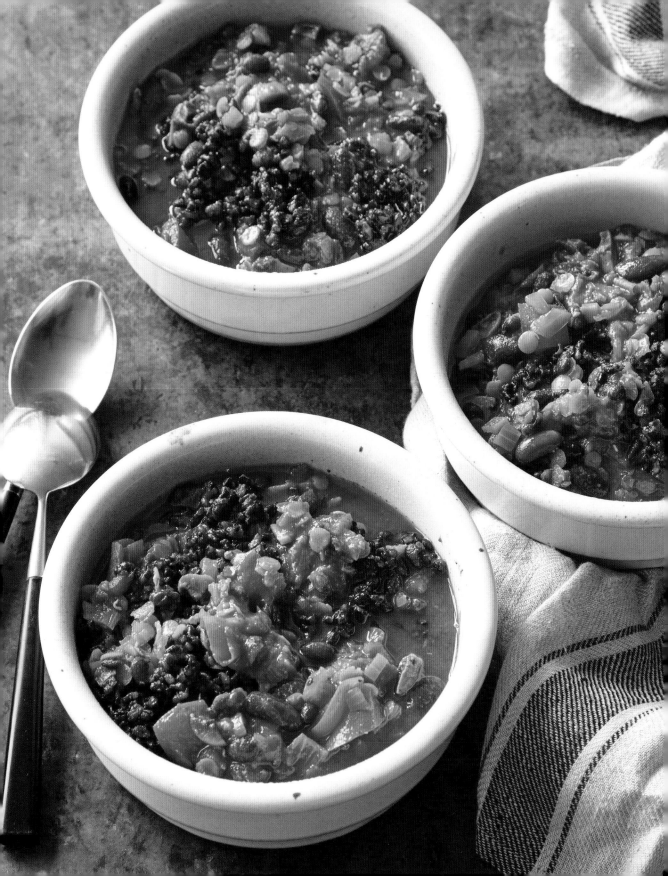

CHAMPION VEGETABLE CHILI

MAKES: *4* (2-CUP) SERVINGS · DIFFICULTY: *easy*

Here's another excellent chili variety that can be served in many ways. Try this over baked and mashed sweet potato; brown, black, or red rice; quinoa; or greens greens greens. Use it as a filling in a collard wrap. Let us know what other creative ways you come up with to enjoy this dish!

1½ cups Vegetable Broth (page 6)

1 red onion, chopped

½ cup minced celery

2 to 3 cups chopped mushrooms (any kind)

1 red bell pepper, seeded and chopped

1 zucchini, chopped

1 small hot chili pepper, seeded and finely minced (optional)

2 garlic cloves, minced

3 tablespoons jarred tomato paste

2 tablespoons chili powder, or to taste

1 ¼-inch piece fresh turmeric, grated (or ¼ teaspoon ground)

1 14.5-ounce BPA-free can or Tetra Pak salt-free diced tomatoes, undrained

3 cups cooked or 2 15.5-ounce BPA-free cans or Tetra Paks pinto beans, drained and rinsed

1 cup corn kernels

2 teaspoons Savory Spice Blend (page 4), or to taste

½ teaspoon smoked paprika

In a large pot, heat 1 cup of the broth over medium heat. Add the onion and celery and cook until softened, about 5 minutes. Add the mushrooms, bell pepper, zucchini, chili (if using), and garlic and cook until softened, stirring occasionally, about 10 minutes. Stir in the tomato paste, chili powder, and turmeric; then add the tomatoes, pinto beans, and remaining ½ cup of broth. Simmer until the vegetables are tender, stirring occasionally, about 45 minutes. Add a little water if the chili gets too thick to your liking. Stir in the corn, Savory Spice Blend, and paprika. Serve hot.

Daily Dozen Foods

✗ BEANS   ✗ OTHER VEGETABLES   ✗ HERBS AND SPICES

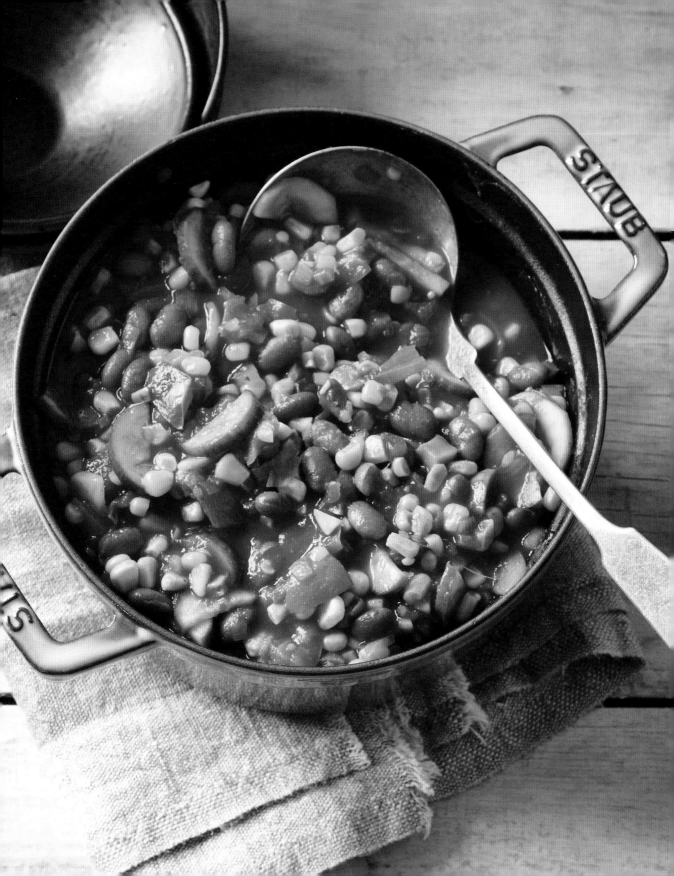

FIVE

SALADS AND DRESSINGS

You won't find any recipes in this cookbook for a side salad of iceberg lettuce with a few carrot shavings and half a cherry tomato, mayonnaise-laden macaroni salad, or any other so-called salad that's virtually devoid of taste and nutrition. The salads in this chapter are rich with flavor and crunch, and can be served as your entrée, a starter, a side, or even a snack. And, with so much added goodness, including nuts, seeds, and fruits, you'll keep busy ticking off lots of the Daily Dozen checkboxes.

GOLDEN QUINOA TABOULI

KALE SALAD WITH AVOCADO
GODDESS DRESSING

BLACK BEAN GAZPACHO SALAD

SESAME PURPLE CABBAGE &
CARROT SLAW

CHOPPED VEGETABLE SALAD

MANGO-AVOCADO-KALE SALAD WITH
GINGER-SESAME ORANGE DRESSING

SUPER SALAD WITH GARLIC CAESAR
DRESSING & HEMP HEARTS

PISTACHIO-SPINACH SALAD WITH
STRAWBERRY BALSAMIC DRESSING

GOLDEN QUINOA TABOULI

MAKES: *6* (1½-CUP) SERVINGS · DIFFICULTY: *easy*

Turmeric adds a touch of gold to the quinoa in this tasty riff on tabouli. More than fifty clinical trials have tested turmeric against a variety of diseases, including lung and brain diseases and a variety of cancers. It's been shown to make colon polyps disappear, speed recovery after surgery, and treat rheumatoid arthritis better than the leading drug. Turmeric also appears to be effective in treating osteoarthritis and other inflammatory conditions, such as lupus and inflammatory bowel disease. I recommend a quarter-teaspoon a day.

1 cup quinoa, washed well, rinsed, and drained

1 ¼-inch piece fresh turmeric, grated (or ¼ teaspoon ground)

DRESSING

2 tablespoons blended peeled lemon (see page 3)

1 tablespoon Date Syrup (page 3)

1½ teaspoons Savory Spice Blend (page 4)

SALAD

1½ cups cooked or 1 15.5-ounce BPA-free can or Tetra Pak salt-free chickpeas, drained and rinsed

2 Roma tomatoes, chopped

1 small ripe Hass avocado, peeled, pitted, and diced

1 cup chopped cucumber

½ cup minced fresh parsley, mint, or cilantro

2 scallions, minced

Ground black pepper

4 cups torn salad greens (my favorite is baby arugula), to serve

In a saucepan, bring 1¾ cups of water to a boil. Add the quinoa and turmeric and reduce the heat to low. Cover and simmer until the water is absorbed, about 15 minutes. Drain well to remove any excess moisture. Transfer the quinoa to a large bowl and set aside to cool.

DRESSING: In a small bowl, combine the lemon, Date Syrup, Savory Spice Blend, and 3 tablespoons of water.

SALAD: When the quinoa is cool, add the chickpeas, tomatoes, avocado, cucumber, parsley, and scallions. Pour on the dressing and season with black pepper to taste. Mix gently to combine. Cover and refrigerate for at least 1 hour, or until ready to serve. The tabouli tastes best if enjoyed on the same day it is made. To serve, spoon over torn salad greens.

10 WAYS TO GET YOUR DAILY TURMERIC

1. Add it to a smoothie.
2. Use it in curries (page 130).
3. Add it to grain dishes (page 140).
4. Blend it into salad dressings.
5. Add it to pasta dishes.
6. Mash it into a baked sweet potato.
7. Add it to soups.
8. Sprinkle it on your oatmeal.
9. Blend it into bean spreads.
10. Add it to your pumpkin pie.

Daily Dozen Foods

X BEANS   X GREENS   X OTHER VEGETABLES   X HERBS AND SPICES   X WHOLE GRAINS

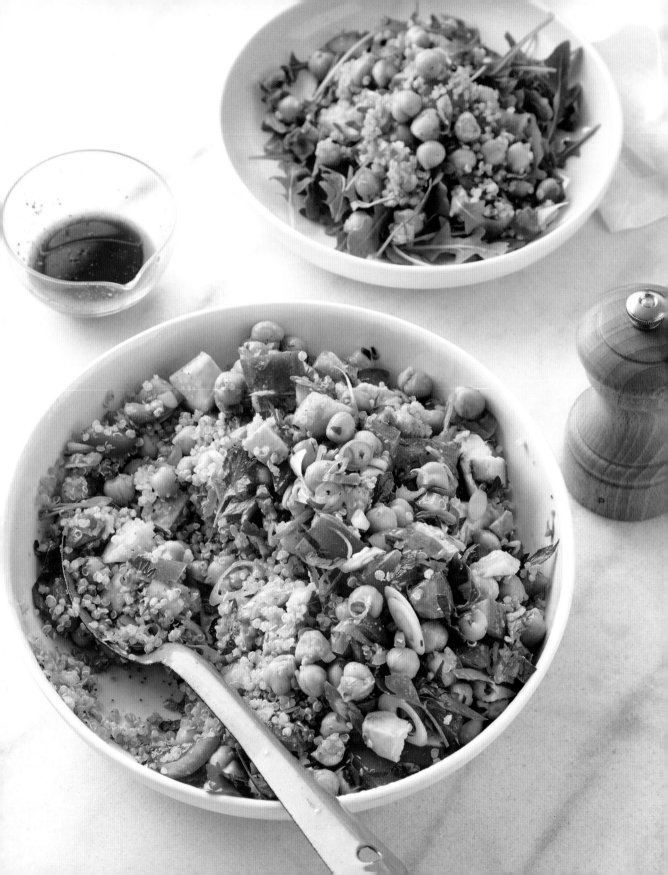

KALE SALAD WITH
AVOCADO GODDESS DRESSING

MAKES: *4* (2½-CUP) SERVINGS · DIFFICULTY: *easy*

Is there anything kale cannot do?

DRESSING

1 small ripe Hass avocado, peeled and pitted

1 scallion, coarsely chopped

1 garlic clove, crushed

¼ cup chopped fresh parsley

1 tablespoon minced fresh tarragon, or 1 teaspoon dried

2 tablespoons rice vinegar

2 teaspoons blended peeled lemon (see page 3)

1 tablespoon nutritional yeast

1 teaspoon Date Syrup (page 3)

½ teaspoon white miso paste

½ teaspoon Savory Spice Blend (page 4), or to taste

SALAD

4 small or medium beets, trimmed and scrubbed

1 bunch red kale, washed, tough stems removed

1½ cups cooked or 1 15.5-ounce BPA-free can or Tetra Pak salt-free black beans, drained and rinsed

¼ cup raw walnuts, or other nut

DRESSING: In a blender or food processor, combine all the ingredients for the dressing and blend well, scraping down the sides as needed, until smooth. If the dressing is too thick for your liking, add up to ⅓ cup of water and blend to incorporate. Taste to adjust the seasonings. Transfer the dressing to a container with a tight-fitting lid and refrigerate until ready to serve.

SALAD: Preheat the oven to 425°F. Arrange the beets in a baking dish, cover, and bake until tender, 40 to 60 minutes, depending on the size of the beets. Remove from the oven, uncover, and allow to cool. When cool enough to handle, remove the skins from the beets, if desired. (They should slip off easily.) Slice, dice, or quarter the beets and transfer to a large bowl. Finely chop the kale and add to the bowl. Add the black beans and walnuts. Toss gently to combine. When ready to serve, toss the salad with as much of the dressing as desired.

TIP: The Avocado Goddess Dressing is also great over roasted sweet potatoes and steamed cauliflower.

Daily Dozen Foods

X BEANS   X GREENS   X OTHER VEGETABLES   X NUTS AND SEEDS   X HERBS AND SPICES

VINEGAR

Hello. My name is Michael, and I am a vinegar-aholic. Yes. I have an entire bar stocked with vinegars with different flavors to complement different dishes. I put strawberry vinegars on peaches, chocolate vinegar on fresh strawberries, smoky vinegar on savory entrées, peach vinegar on mangoes, and, yes, mango vinegar on peaches. When people think of vinegar, distilled white vinegar may pop into their mind, but that belongs under the sink with other natural cleaners, not the pantry. The science on the benefits of vinegars inspired me to explore this surprisingly exotic and far-reaching world, and I'm so glad it did. I try to be a really frugal person, but the three things I splurge on are blazing-fast Internet service, fresh dates every fall, and exotic vinegars.

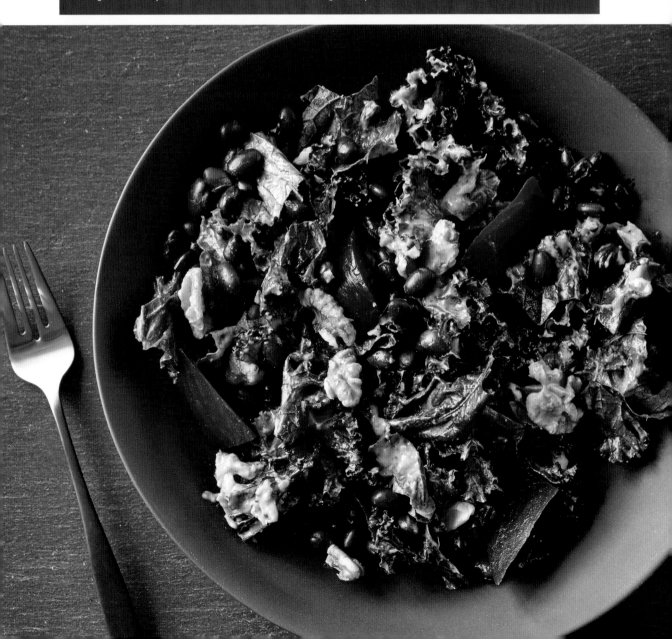

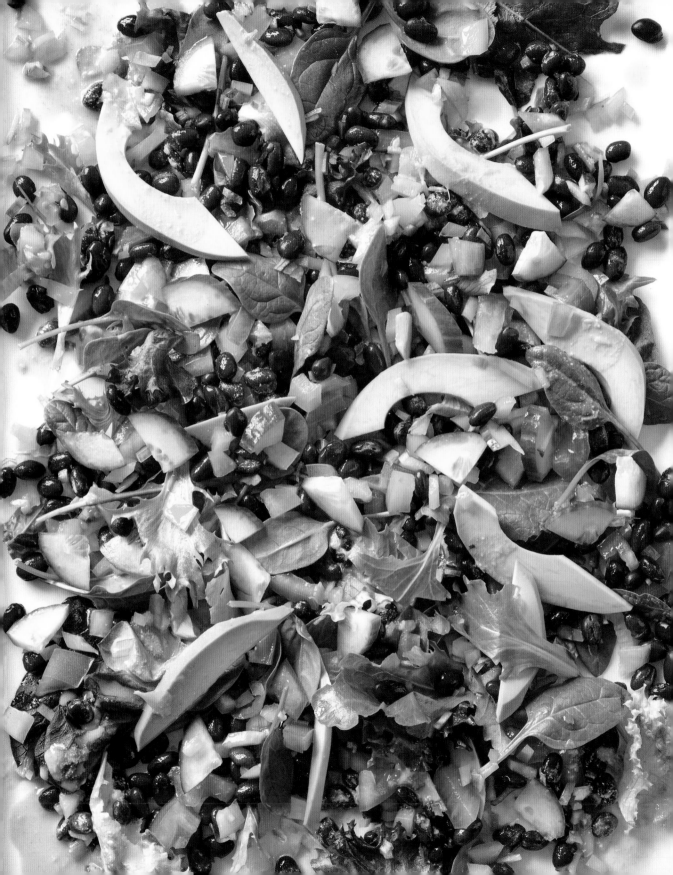

BLACK BEAN GAZPACHO SALAD

MAKES: *4* (2-CUP) SERVINGS · DIFFICULTY: *easy*

I knew beans were healthy, but I didn't realize just how healthy until all the amazing microbiome research started coming out. I encourage you to get into the (delicious) habit of eating legumes throughout the day. Before I started pressure-cooking my own, I always kept an open can of beans in the fridge as a reminder to put them in anything and everything, such as this salad, which, taking its cue from the famous chilled soup, features gazpacho ingredients with black beans and a zesty dressing served over greens.

DRESSING

1 teaspoon white miso paste

2 teaspoons blended peeled lime (see page 3)

1 tablespoon nutritional yeast

¼ teaspoon ground cumin, or to taste

SALAD

1½ cups cooked or 1 15.5-ounce BPA-free can or Tetra Pak salt-free black beans, drained and rinsed

1 ripe tomato, seeded and finely chopped

1 red or yellow bell pepper, chopped

1 cup chopped cucumber

¼ cup minced red onion

1 garlic clove, minced

1 teaspoon minced jalapeño pepper

5 cups mixed salad greens

1 small ripe Hass avocado

Healthy Hot Sauce (page 8) (optional)

DRESSING: In a small bowl, combine all the dressing ingredients and stir to blend well. Set aside.

SALAD: In a large bowl, combine the black beans, tomato, bell pepper, cucumber, onion, garlic, and jalapeño.

Pour the dressing over the salad and toss lightly. Cover and set aside for 30 minutes, or refrigerate overnight.

Divide the salad greens among individual salad plates and top with the black bean gazpacho. Halve and pit the avocado and cut it into ½-inch dice. Top the salads with the avocado and Healthy Hot Sauce (if using). Serve at once.

Daily Dozen Foods

✗ BEANS ✗ GREENS ✗ OTHER VEGETABLES ✗ HERBS AND SPICES

SESAME PURPLE CABBAGE & CARROT SLAW

MAKES: *4* (1¼-CUP) SERVINGS · DIFFICULTY: *easy*

I always keep purple cabbage in the fridge. It's cheap, colorful, and cruciferocious. And, it seems to keep forever, not that it's ever lasted long enough in my household for us to find out. This vibrant slaw is a nice, much more flavorful change from the typical heavy, mayonnaise-covered coleslaw—and way better for you!

DRESSING

2 tablespoons tahini

2 tablespoons rice vinegar

2 teaspoons blended peeled lemon (see page 3)

2 teaspoons Date Syrup (page 3)

1 teaspoon grated fresh ginger

1 teaspoon white miso paste

SLAW

3 cups shredded purple cabbage

1 large carrot, grated

12 snow peas, cut diagonally into thin matchsticks

2 scallions, minced

1 cup red grapes, halved

2 tablespoons chopped fresh cilantro (optional)

2 tablespoons sesame seeds

DRESSING: In a small bowl, combine all of the dressing ingredients with 2 tablespoons of water. Stir well to blend and set aside.

SLAW: In a large bowl, combine the cabbage, carrot, snow peas, scallions, grapes, and cilantro (if using). Pour on the dressing and toss gently to coat. Taste and adjust the seasoning as desired. Sprinkle with the sesame seeds. Refrigerate, covered, until ready to serve.

CABBAGE

Antioxidants are your body's defense squad, charged with destroying DNA-damaging free radicals. No need to buy some exotic, so-called superfruit to get them, though. According to a USDA database of common foods, red and purple cabbage provide some of the highest levels of antioxidants per dollar.[110] In fact, purple cabbages may have nearly three times the antioxidant power per dollar than do blueberries.[111]

Daily Dozen Foods

✗ OTHER FRUITS   ✗ CRUCIFEROUS VEGETABLES   ✗ OTHER VEGETABLES   ✗ NUTS AND SEEDS   ✗ HERBS AND SPICES

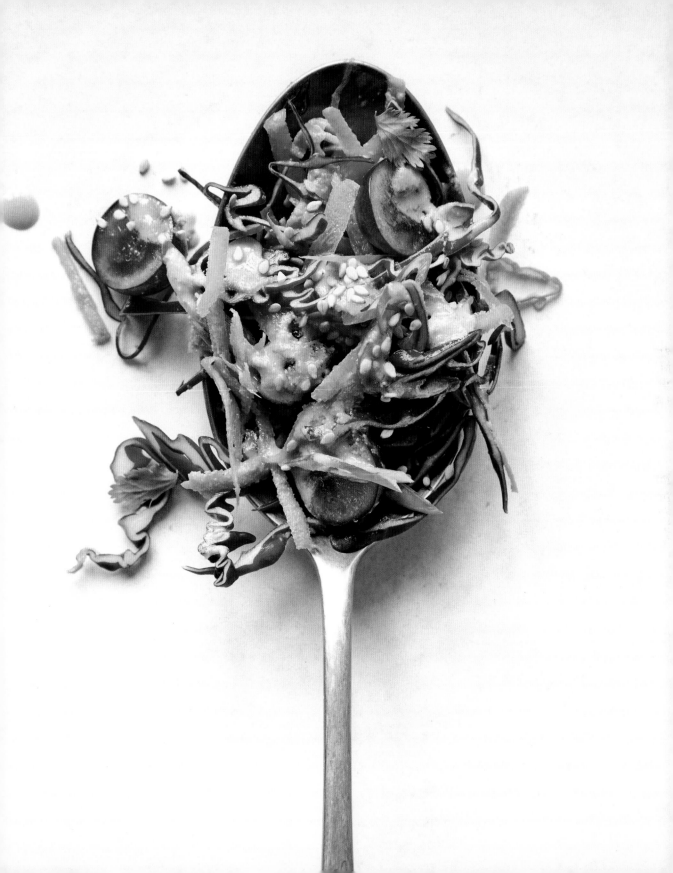

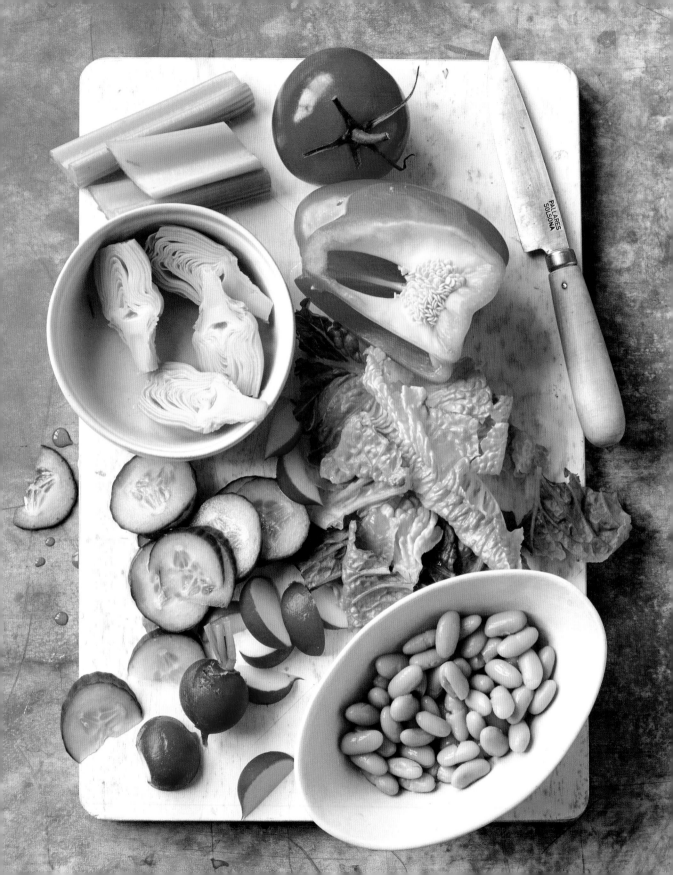

CHOPPED VEGETABLE SALAD

MAKES: *4* (2½-CUP) SERVINGS · DIFFICULTY: *easy*

One of the great things about this recipe is that it's really flexible, so you can cater to whatever you're in the mood for tasting and enjoying. Mix and match ingredients, leaving out any you don't like or may not have on hand and adding other favorites.

1 small head romaine lettuce, chopped into bite-sized pieces

2 radishes, chopped

1 ripe tomato, chopped

1 cup chopped cucumber

½ small orange or red bell pepper, chopped

½ cup chopped celery

3 artichoke hearts, chopped

1½ cups cooked or 1 15.5-ounce BPA-free can or Tetra Pak cannellini beans, drained and rinsed

Ranch Dressing (page 7)

In a large bowl, combine the lettuce, radishes, tomato, cucumber, bell pepper, celery, artichoke hearts, and cannellini beans.

Drizzle the Ranch Dressing onto the salad and toss to combine.

DIY SALAD BAR

Keep a selection of salad ingredients prepped so your own personal salad bar is ready whenever you get a craving. Wash and spin-dry salad greens; mix up a few of the dressings in this chapter; and keep a variety of washed, sliced, and diced veggies in tightly covered containers so all you have to do is create your salad masterpiece. Keep handy pantry ingredient add-ins, such as nuts and dried fruit. For variety, change up the greens you use in salads, try different vinegars in the dressings, and add new fruit, veggie, and nut combos.

Daily Dozen Foods

✗ BEANS   ✗ GREENS   ✗ OTHER VEGETABLES   ✗ NUTS AND SEEDS   ✗ HERBS AND SPICES

MANGO-AVOCADO-KALE SALAD WITH GINGER-SESAME ORANGE DRESSING

MAKES: *4* SERVINGS · DIFFICULTY: *easy*

Mangoes are one of my favorite fruits. I just love their taste and texture. But I've recently discovered a new fruit I love even more—the pawpaw, North America's largest native fruit. They aren't available in stores because they're too delicate, but keep an eye out for local pawpaw festivals and ask about them at your farmers' market. If you're lucky enough to find a pawpaw, you can use it in this salad instead of mango.

DRESSING

½ orange, peeled

1 tablespoon rice vinegar

2 tablespoons tahini

1½ teaspoons grated fresh ginger

1 garlic clove, minced

1 tablespoon minced scallion

2 teaspoons minced fresh parsley or cilantro

1 teaspoon white miso paste

1 teaspoon Date Syrup (page 3)

1 (¼-inch) piece fresh turmeric, grated, or ¼ teaspoon ground turmeric

⅛ teaspoon cayenne pepper (optional)

SALAD

5 cups chopped red kale or baby spinach leaves

1 ripe mango, peeled, pitted, and cut into ½-inch dice

1 ripe Hass avocado, peeled, pitted, and cut into ½-inch dice

DRESSING: In a mini-blender or small food processor, combine all the dressing ingredients and blend until smooth. Set aside.

SALAD: In a large bowl, combine the kale, mango, and avocado. Pour on as much of the dressing as desired and toss gently to combine.

NOTE: If you don't have a mini-blender or small food processor, you may want to double the dressing recipe to make in a larger machine (and then save half for another day).

Daily Dozen Foods

✗ OTHER FRUITS   ✗ GREENS   ✗ NUTS AND SEEDS   ✗ HERBS AND SPICES

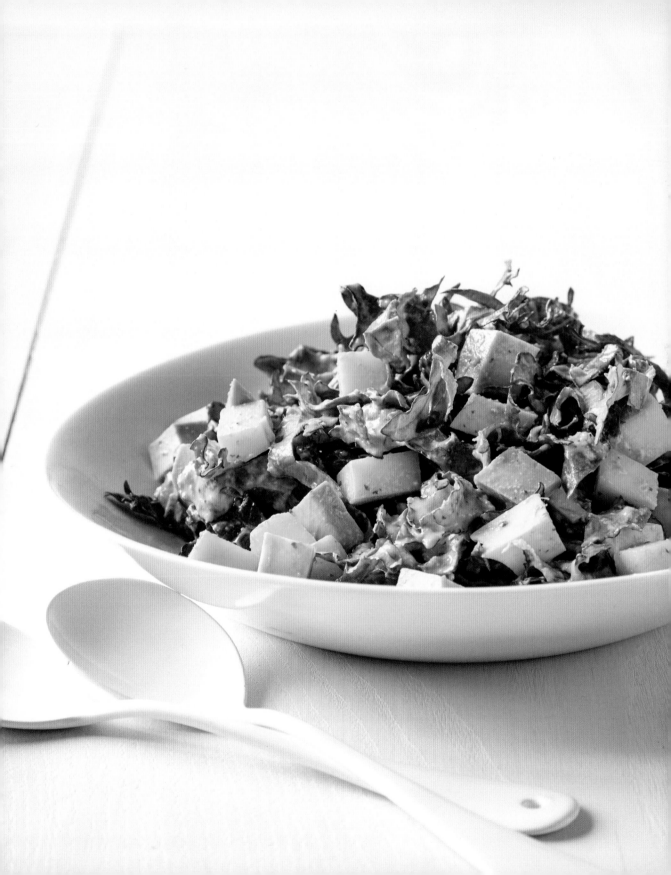

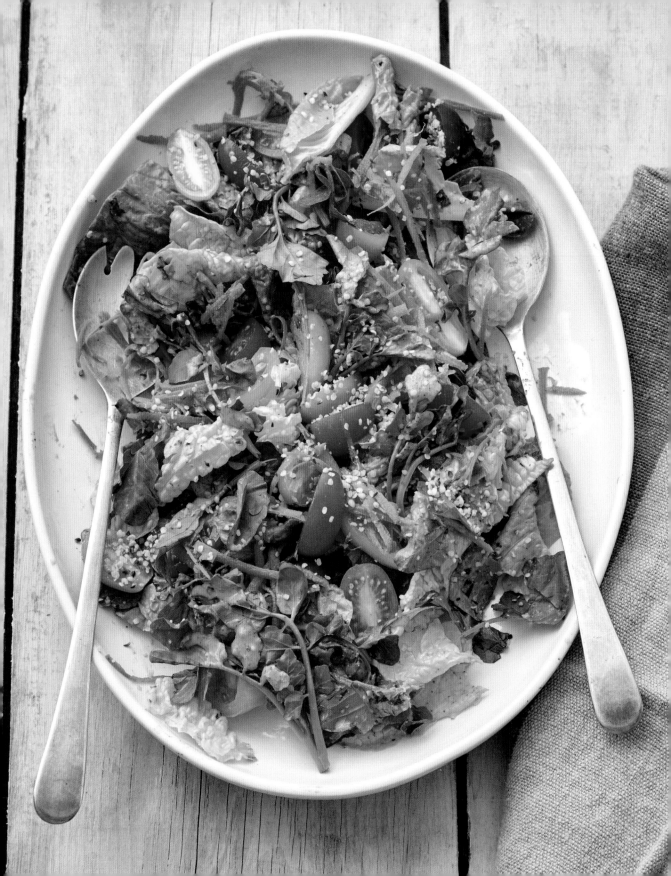

SUPER SALAD WITH GARLIC CAESAR DRESSING & HEMP HEARTS

MAKES: *4* (3-CUP) SERVINGS · DIFFICULTY: *easy*

Add bite-sized dices of steamed or sautéed tempeh to this salad for a pretty perfect entrée.

DRESSING

2 garlic cloves, crushed

2 tablespoons nutritional yeast

1 tablespoon almond butter

1 tablespoon blended peeled lemon (see page 3)

1 tablespoon white miso paste

1 tablespoon minced fresh parsley

1 teaspoon salt-free stone-ground mustard

1 ¼-inch piece fresh turmeric, grated (or ¼ teaspoon ground)

1 teaspoon Savory Spice Blend (page 4), or to taste

SALAD

1 head romaine lettuce, trimmed and torn into small pieces

1 bunch watercress, stemmed and chopped, or 2 cups baby spinach

1 cup halved cherry or grape tomatoes

1 carrot, shredded

3 tablespoons hulled hemp seeds (hemp hearts)

DRESSING: In a blender, combine ½ cup of water with all the dressing ingredients and blend until smooth. Taste and adjust the seasoning to your liking. Set aside.

SALAD: In a large bowl, combine all the salad ingredients, toss lightly with the dressing, and serve.

Daily Dozen Foods

✗ GREENS   ✗ OTHER VEGETABLES   ✗ NUTS AND SEEDS   ✗ HERBS AND SPICES

PISTACHIO-SPINACH SALAD WITH STRAWBERRY BALSAMIC DRESSING

MAKES: *4* (2¼-CUP) SERVINGS · DIFFICULTY: *easy*

This fancy-looking salad is incredibly easy to make. If fresh strawberries are unavailable, substitute frozen berries that have been thawed to room temperature. (Half our freezer is stocked with frozen berries, and the other half with frozen greens!)

DRESSING

1 cup strawberries, hulled and halved

1 tablespoon chopped shallot

¼ cup balsamic vinegar

1 tablespoon Date Syrup (page 3)

½ teaspoon salt-free stone-ground mustard

1 teaspoon fresh thyme, or ½ teaspoon dried

½ teaspoon poppy seeds

¼ teaspoon ground black pepper

SALAD

8 cups baby spinach

½ cucumber, halved and thinly sliced

¼ cup raw pistachios

DRESSING: In a blender, combine the strawberries, shallot, vinegar, Date Syrup, mustard, and thyme. Blend until smooth. Stir in the poppy seeds and black pepper and set aside.

SALAD: In a large bowl, combine all the salad ingredients, dress to your liking, and toss lightly to coat.

Daily Dozen Foods

✗ BERRIES   ✗ GREENS   ✗ OTHER VEGETABLES   ✗ NUTS AND SEEDS   ✗ HERBS AND SPICES

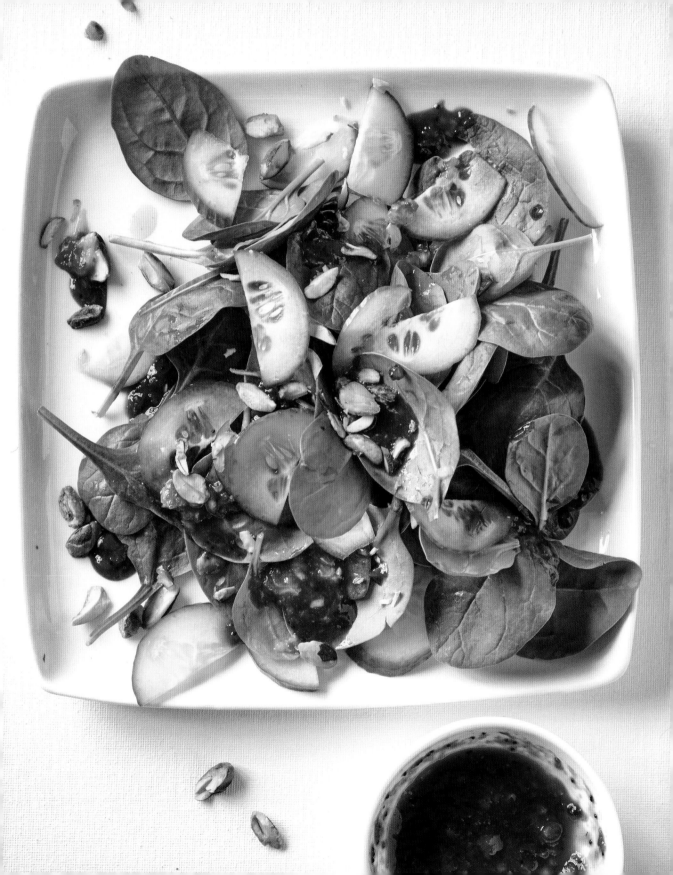

BLACK BEAN BURGERS

SLOPPY JACKS

CURRIED CHICKPEA WRAPS

SPINACH & MUSHROOM BLACK BEAN BURRITOS

VERACRUZ TEMPEH LETTUCE WRAPS

BEET BURGERS

BEANS & GREENS QUESADILLAS

SIX

BURGERS, WRAPS, AND MORE

Beets. Black beans. Tempeh. Chickpeas. Teff. Jackfruit.
The recipes in this chapter will introduce you to amazing
flavors bursting from creative takes on traditional dishes.
Say goodbye to artery-clogging burgers!

BLACK BEAN BURGERS

MAKES: *4* SERVINGS · DIFFICULTY: *easy*

There can never be enough ways to get beans into your daily meals. This is one of the best. Serve on toasted 100% whole-grain bread with all the fixings. These burgers freeze well, so consider doubling the recipe so you'll have them ready for just-thaw-and-indulge moments.

1 cup old-fashioned rolled oats

½ cup walnut pieces

1 ¼-inch piece fresh turmeric, grated (or ¼ teaspoon ground)

½ cup chopped red onion

⅓ cup chopped mushrooms

1½ cups cooked or 1 15-ounce BPA-free can or Tetra Pak salt-free black beans, well rinsed and drained

2 tablespoons tahini or almond butter

1 tablespoon ground flaxseeds

1 tablespoon nutritional yeast

1 tablespoon chopped fresh parsley

2 teaspoons white miso paste

1 teaspoon onion powder

½ teaspoon garlic powder

½ teaspoon smoked paprika

1 teaspoon Savory Spice Blend (page 4)

Pulse the oats, walnuts, and turmeric in a food processor until they are finely ground. Add the onion, mushrooms, beans, tahini, and flaxseeds and pulse until well combined. Add the remaining ingredients and pulse to mix well.

Pinch some of the mixture between your thumb and index finger to test whether it holds together. If the mixture is too wet, add more oats. If the mixture is too dry, add a little water, 1 tablespoon at a time. Transfer the mixture to a work surface and divide into four equal portions. Shape each into a patty about ½-inch thick and transfer to a plate. Refrigerate for 30 minutes.

Preheat the oven to 375°F.

Line a baking sheet with a silicone mat or parchment paper and arrange the burgers on it. Bake until hot and lightly browned, turning once, about 25 minutes. Serve hot, as desired.

Daily Dozen Foods

✗ BEANS   ✗ OTHER VEGETABLES   ✗ FLAXSEEDS   ✗ NUTS AND SEEDS   ✗ HERBS AND SPICES   ✗ WHOLE GRAINS

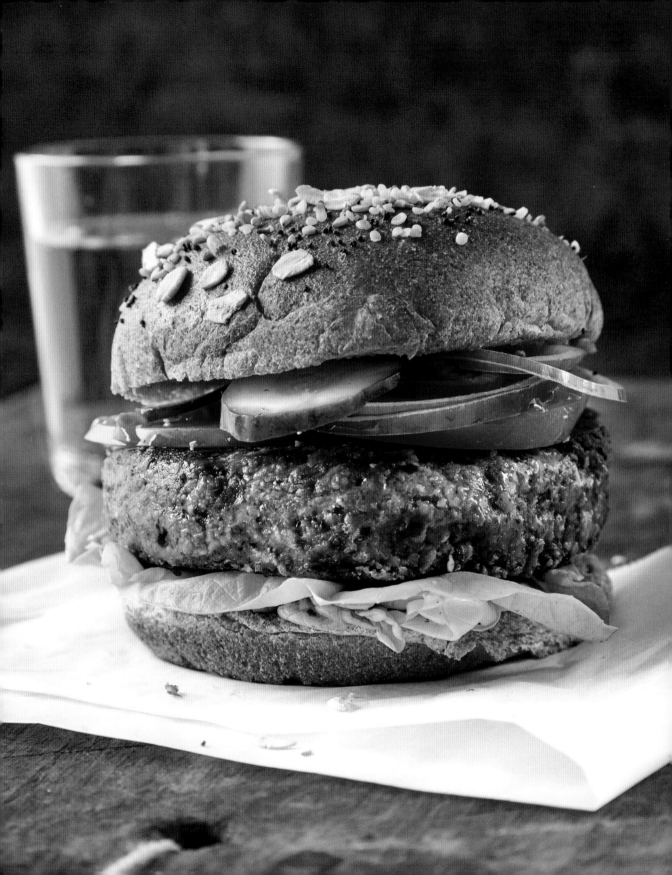

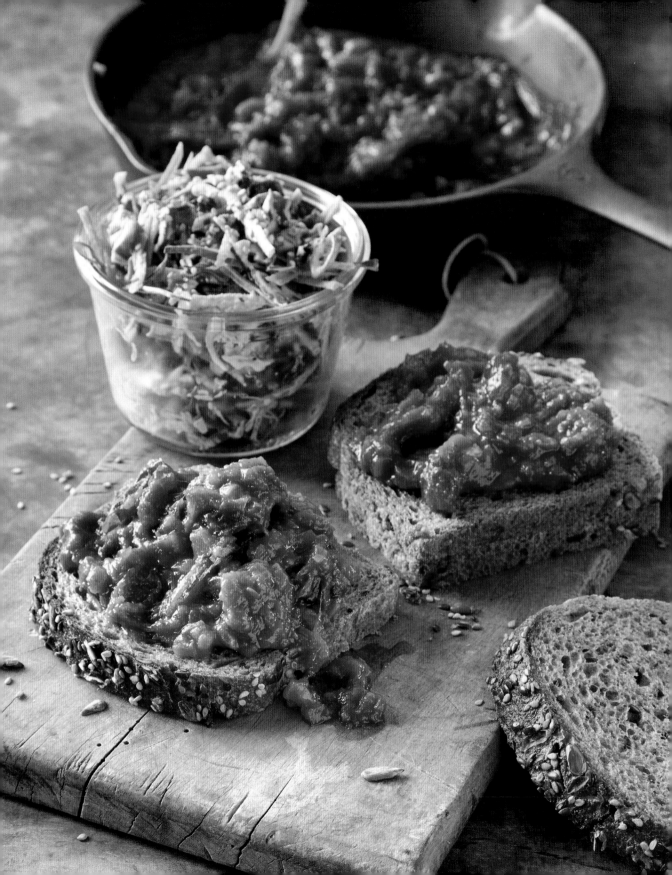

SLOPPY JACKS

MAKES: *4* SERVINGS (ABOUT 1 CUP FILLING PER SANDWICH) · DIFFICULTY: *easy*

Jackfruit is native to Southern Asia and has been cultivated for as long as six thousand years. Despite its popularity and long culinary history overseas, it's just starting to make a name for itself in the United States because of its versatile texture and interesting flavor—a mix of mango, banana, apple, and pineapple. Jackfruit is low in calories and fat, and rich in fiber. You may be able to find fresh jackfruit in Asian markets, or you can just buy it canned, as I normally do.

---

1 20-ounce BPA-free can jackfruit (packed in water, not syrup), drained and rinsed

1 tablespoon nutritional yeast

1 teaspoon Savory Spice Blend (page 4)

½ teaspoon smoked paprika

½ teaspoon chili powder

1 small red onion, minced

½ red bell pepper, seeded and minced

¾ cup jarred or Tetra Pak salt-free tomato purée

2 tablespoons date sugar

1 tablespoon salt-free stone-ground mustard

4 slices 100% whole-grain bread

Blot the drained and rinsed jackfruit dry with paper towels or a clean kitchen towel. Remove and discard any hard pieces of its core. Transfer the jackfruit to a bowl and add the nutritional yeast, Savory Spice Blend, paprika, and chili powder. Toss to coat and set aside.

Heat ½ cup of water in a large skillet over medium heat. Add the onion and bell pepper, cover, and cook until soft, about 5 minutes. Stir in the tomato purée, date sugar, and mustard. Add the coated jackfruit and reduce the heat to low. Cover and simmer for 25 to 30 minutes, stirring frequently, adding a little more water, 1 tablespoon at a time, if needed so the mixture doesn't stick to the skillet. As the jackfruit cooks, use two forks to shred it into smaller pieces. Cook uncovered for the final 5 minutes to thicken the sauce. To serve, spoon the jackfruit mixture onto the bread and serve hot.

Daily Dozen Foods

✗ OTHER FRUITS   ✗ OTHER VEGETABLES   ✗ HERBS AND SPICES   ✗ WHOLE GRAINS

CURRIED CHICKPEA WRAPS

MAKES: *4* WRAPS (1 CUP FILLING PER WRAP) · DIFFICULTY: *easy*

One of the ingredients of curry powder, which is one of my favorite spice mixes, is turmeric. Besides being so good for you, turmeric gives the blend its beautiful yellow color. The curried chickpea filling in this recipe is also great in lettuce wraps or served as a dip. Try it with Three-Seed Crackers (page 34) for a flavorful starter or snack.

1½ cups cooked or 1 15.5-ounce BPA-free can or Tetra Pak salt-free chickpeas, drained and rinsed

1½ teaspoons curry powder, or to taste

1 teaspoon blended peeled lemon (see page 3)

1 teaspoon date sugar

¼ teaspoon white miso paste

Savory Spice Blend (page 4)

½ cup chopped celery

⅓ cup shredded carrot

⅓ cup chopped cashews

⅓ cup raisins

1 firm sweet apple, cored and chopped

1 tablespoon chopped scallion

4 100% whole-grain tortillas

2 cups shredded lettuce

In a food processor, combine 1 cup of the chickpeas with the curry powder, lemon, date sugar, miso, and Savory Spice Blend to taste with 3 to 4 tablespoons of water. Process until smooth. Add the remaining ½ cup of chickpeas and the celery, carrot, cashews, raisins, apple, and scallion, and pulse just to combine and break up the chickpeas a bit. Taste and adjust the seasonings, if needed.

To assemble, divide the chickpea mixture evenly onto the tortillas and top each with the lettuce. Tightly roll up each of the tortillas to make a wrap. Cut each wrap in half and serve immediately.

CHICKPEAS

The more chickpeas (and other legumes) you eat, the healthier you are. In one study, researchers divided overweight subjects into two groups. The first group was asked to eat 5 cups a week of chickpeas, lentils, split peas, or navy beans—but not to change their diet in any other way. The second group was asked to simply cut out 500 calories a day from their diet. Guess who got healthier? The group directed to eat *more* food. Eating chickpeas and other beans was shown to be just as effective at slimming waistlines and improving blood sugar control as it is at cutting calories. The legume group also gained additional benefits in the form of improved cholesterol and insulin regulation.[112]

Daily Dozen Foods

✗ BEANS   ✗ OTHER FRUITS   ✗ GREENS   ✗ OTHER VEGETABLES   ✗ NUTS AND SEEDS   ✗ HERBS AND SPICES   ✗ WHOLE GRAINS

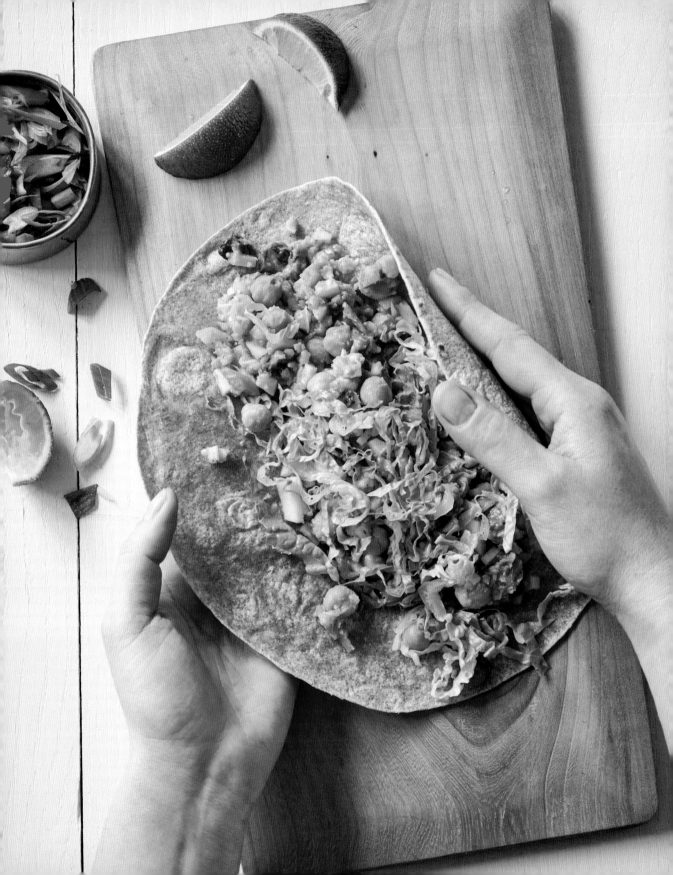

SPINACH & MUSHROOM BLACK BEAN BURRITOS

MAKES: *4* SERVINGS · DIFFICULTY: *easy*

Spinach is not my favorite green. I love all dark green leafies, but I'm more likely to go for a cruciferous one, such as kale or arugula. Spinach is a great option for newbies, though. It doesn't have a strong distinctive flavor, so you can blend handfuls into a smoothie and hardly taste it. Spinach also fits well into foods like burritos, such as this nutritious one featuring mushrooms and black beans. This filling is so good you shouldn't save it only for burritos. Make a double batch so you have it on hand to heat and eat whenever and however you want.

1½ cups cooked or 1 15.5-ounce BPA-free can or Tetra Pak salt-free black beans, drained and rinsed

½ cup minced red onion

2 garlic cloves, minced

2 cups chopped mushrooms

4 cups baby spinach

1 tablespoon nutritional yeast

Savory Spice Blend (page 4)

Cayenne pepper

Healthy Hot Sauce (page 8)

4 100% whole-grain tortillas

Summer Salsa (page 41)

In a bowl, mash the black beans with a fork or potato ricer and set aside.

Heat ¼ cup of water in a skillet and add the onion and garlic. Cook, stirring occasionally, until softened, about 5 minutes. Stir in the mushrooms and cook for 3 minutes longer to soften. Add the spinach and cook, stirring, until the spinach is wilted. Add the mashed black beans and continue to cook, stirring, until the liquid is absorbed. Stir in the nutritional yeast, Savory Spice Blend, cayenne, and hot sauce to taste. Taste and adjust the seasonings to your liking.

To serve, spoon a quarter of the filling down the center of each tortilla. Add more hot sauce, if desired, and roll up each burrito, tucking in the sides as you do so. Serve immediately or, one at a time, place each filled burrito in a hot nonstick skillet for a minute or two—just long enough to lightly brown the outside of the tortillas. Serve with the Summer Salsa.

Daily Dozen Foods

✗ BEANS   ✗ GREENS   ✗ OTHER VEGETABLES   ✗ HERBS AND SPICES   ✗ WHOLE GRAINS

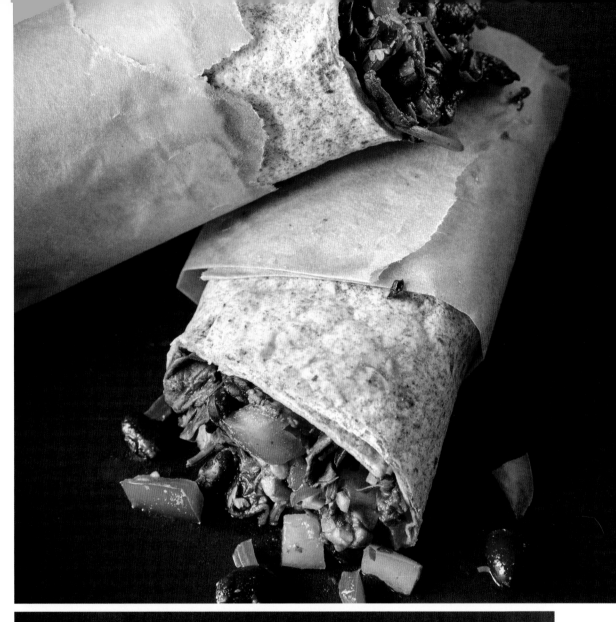

SPINACH

Popeye was right when he bragged he was strong to the finish because he ate his spinach. Of all the food groups analyzed by a team of Harvard University researchers, greens turned out to be associated with the strongest protection against major chronic diseases,[113] including up to about a 20 percent reduction in risk for both heart attacks[114] and strokes[115] associated with every additional daily serving. Comparing spinach, Boston lettuce, endive, radicchio, and romaine lettuce, Cornell University researchers found that spinach was best at suppressing the growth of breast cancer, brain tumor, kidney cancer, lung cancer, pediatric brain tumor, pancreatic cancer, prostate cancer, and stomach cancer cells in vitro.[116]

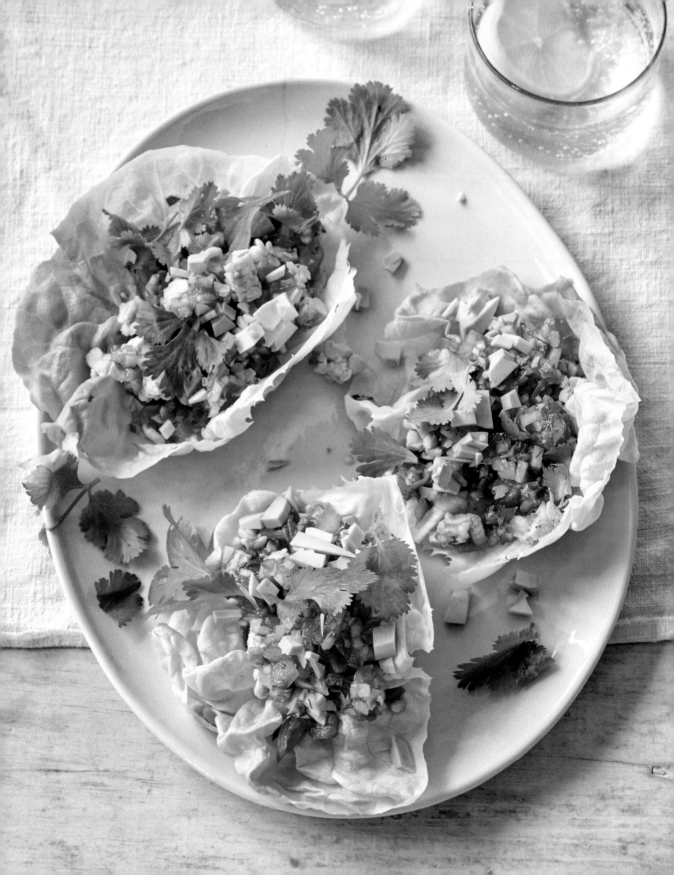

VERACRUZ TEMPEH LETTUCE WRAPS

MAKES: *4* SERVINGS (2 WRAPS PER SERVING) · DIFFICULTY: *moderate*

Nori flakes help give these crunchy wraps a taste of the sea. Look for nori and other sea vegetables in natural food stores, Asian markets, or online.

8 ounces tempeh, cut into ¼-inch dice

2 teaspoons chili powder

2 teaspoons ground cumin

½ teaspoon cayenne pepper

1 small red onion, chopped

2 garlic cloves, minced

1 or 2 jalapeño peppers, seeded and minced

3 Roma tomatoes, chopped

1 teaspoon nori or dulse flakes

1 tablespoon blended peeled lime (see page 3)

8 large romaine or butter lettuce leaves, for wraps

1 ripe Hass avocado, peeled, pitted, and chopped

½ cup chopped fresh cilantro (optional)

Healthy Hot Sauce (page 8) or Summer Salsa (page 41) (optional)

Steam the tempeh in a steamer basket over boiling water for 15 minutes and then set aside, uncovered.

In a shallow bowl, combine the chili powder, cumin, and cayenne; then add the steamed tempeh, tossing lightly to coat.

Heat ¼ cup of water in a skillet over medium-high heat. Add the onion, garlic, and jalapeño and cook for 5 minutes or until soft, adding a little more water if needed so the ingredients don't burn. Stir in the tomatoes and nori and cook until most of the liquid evaporates, about 3 minutes longer. Add the seasoned tempeh and lime and continue to cook until lightly browned, about 4 minutes.

To assemble, spoon some of the filling onto a lettuce leaf and top with some avocado, cilantro (if using), and Healthy Hot Sauce or Summer Salsa to taste (if using). Repeat with the remaining ingredients and serve.

Daily Dozen Foods

X BEANS   X OTHER FRUITS   X GREENS   X OTHER VEGETABLES   X HERBS AND SPICES

BEET BURGERS

MAKES: *6* BURGERS · DIFFICULTY: *moderate*

What's teff? An Ethiopian grain, teff may have been cultivated as many as six thousand years ago. It is tiny—150 grains of teff equal the weight of just a single grain of wheat. The word comes from an Ethiopian root that means "lost," because if you drop a grain of it, you are not likely to find it again. As such, teff cooks more quickly than other grains.

½ cup minced red onion

2 garlic cloves, minced

1 cup finely shredded raw beets

1 cup minced mushrooms

½ teaspoon smoked paprika

½ teaspoon dry mustard (mustard powder)

½ teaspoon ground cumin

½ teaspoon ground coriander

1 ¼-inch piece fresh turmeric, grated (or ¼ teaspoon ground)

1½ cups cooked or 1 15-ounce BPA-free can or Tetra Pak salt-free black beans, rinsed and well drained

1 cup cooked brown, red, or black rice; teff; or quinoa; well drained and blotted dry

1 tablespoon ground flaxseeds

1 tablespoon white miso paste

½ cup old-fashioned rolled oats, ground into coarse flour

½ cup ground walnuts

6 100% whole-grain buns

Heat ¼ cup of water in a large skillet over medium heat. Add the onion and cook until softened, about 5 minutes. Stir in the garlic and then add the beets and mushrooms. Sprinkle on the paprika, mustard, cumin, coriander, and turmeric. Cook until the vegetables are softened and the liquid is absorbed, about 4 minutes.

In a large bowl, mash the beans well to break them up. Add the cooked grain, flaxseeds, and miso. Mash the mixture to combine and then add the oats and walnuts, then the cooked vegetables. Combine until the mixture holds together when pressed between your thumb and forefinger. Divide the mixture into six equal portions and use your hands to shape them into balls. Press the balls into patties and transfer them to a plate. Refrigerate for a minimum of 30 minutes.

Preheat the oven to 375°F. Line a baking sheet with a silicone mat or parchment paper and arrange the burgers on it. Bake for 30 minutes, gently flipping the patties about halfway through. Serve hot with or without a bun and your favorite condiments.

NOTE: Be careful when shredding beets—their bright red color can stain!

SOY

Soybean consumption helps reduce menopausal hot-flash symptoms,[117] as well as decrease a woman's risk of breast cancer.[118] In fact, women diagnosed with breast cancer who ate more soy lived significantly longer and had a significantly lower risk of breast cancer recurrence than those who ate less.[119]

Daily Dozen Foods

✗ BEANS   ✗ OTHER VEGETABLES   ✗ NUTS AND SEEDS   ✗ HERBS AND SPICES   ✗ WHOLE GRAINS

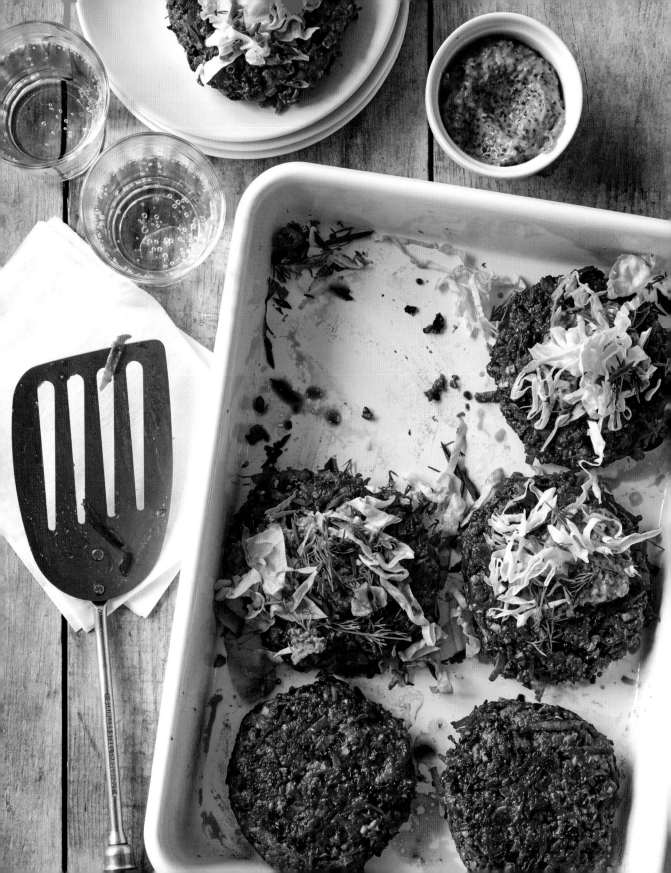

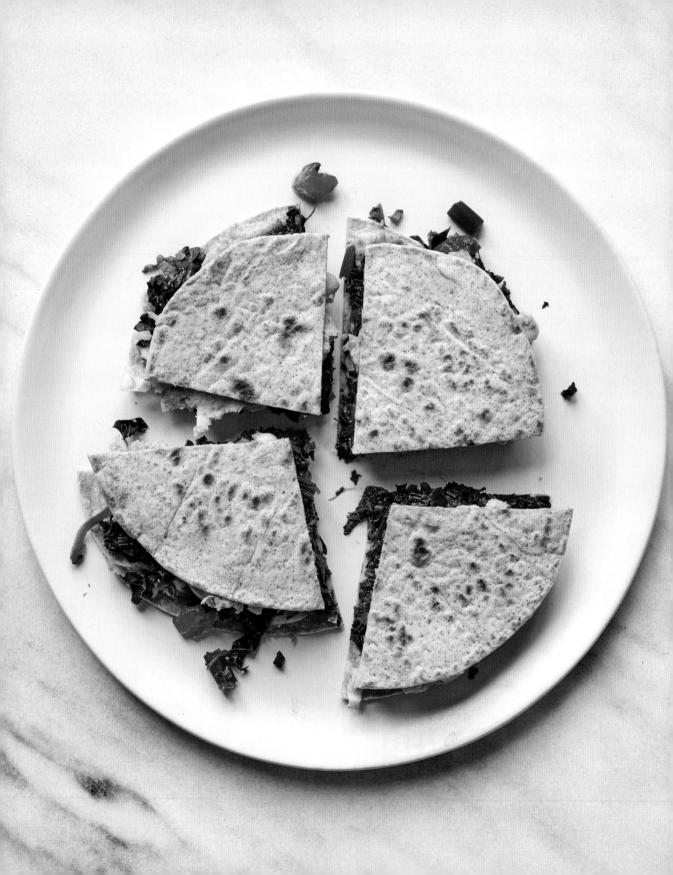

BEANS & GREENS QUESADILLAS

MAKES: *4* SERVINGS · DIFFICULTY: *easy*

Who needs queso when you can enjoy quesadillas filled with a zesty blend of beans and greens?

---

1 small red onion, minced

3 garlic cloves, minced

1 bunch (about 5 cups) chard or red kale, finely chopped

2 Roma tomatoes, chopped

1½ cups cooked or 1 15.5-ounce BPA-free can or Tetra Pak salt-free cannellini beans, drained and rinsed

2 tablespoons nutritional yeast

1 teaspoon chili powder

Savory Spice Blend (page 4) (optional)

Healthy Hot Sauce (page 8) (optional)

4 (10-inch) 100% whole-grain tortillas

Summer Salsa (page 41) (optional)

Heat ¼ cup of water in a pot over medium heat. Add the onion and garlic and cook until softened, about 5 minutes. Add the chard and tomatoes, and continue to cook, stirring, until the greens are tender and the liquid is cooked off, about 5 minutes longer.

While the greens are cooking, mash the beans in a bowl and stir in the nutritional yeast, chili powder, and Savory Spice Blend and Healthy Hot Sauce to taste (if using). Mix well.

Drain off any remaining liquid from the greens mixture and then stir into the bean mixture. Taste and adjust the seasonings, if needed.

Divide the filling among the tortillas, spreading it evenly over the bottom half of each. Fold the top half of the tortilla over the filling, pressing down lightly to hold the halves together. Place two of the quesadillas in a large nonstick skillet or griddle over medium heat. Cook until lightly browned on both sides, turning once, about 3 minutes per side. Repeat with the remaining quesadillas. To serve, cut each quesadilla into three or four wedges and arrange on plates. Serve with Summer Salsa, if desired.

Daily Dozen Foods

✗ BEANS   ✗ GREENS   ✗ OTHER VEGETABLES   ✗ HERBS AND SPICES   ✗ WHOLE GRAINS

SEVEN

VERY VEGGIE MAINS

Thankfully, the days of relegating vegetables to the side of our plates are fading fast and with good reason. Bite for bite, you just can't beat veggies. The dishes in this chapter are innovative, delicious, and the perfect way to spotlight vegetables on center stage!

ZUCCHINI NOODLES WITH
AVOCADO-CASHEW ALFREDO

PESTO CARROT NOODLES WITH
WHITE BEANS & TOMATOES

SPAGHETTI SQUASH ARRABIATA

ROASTED VEGETABLE LASAGNA

STUFFED PORTOBELLOS WITH
HERBED MUSHROOM GRAVY

WHOLE ROASTED CAULIFLOWER
WITH LEMON TAHINI SAUCE

VEGETABLE STACKS WITH
TOMATO-RED PEPPER COULIS

CAULIFLOWER STEAKS
WITH CHERMOULA SAUCE

PORTOBELLOS & GREENS ON TOAST

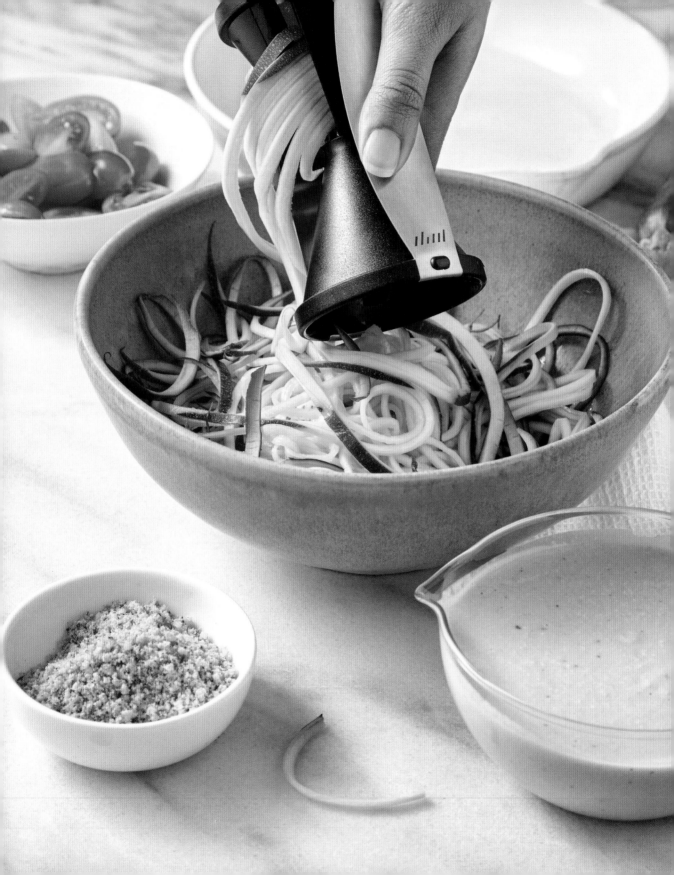

ZUCCHINI NOODLES WITH AVOCADO-CASHEW ALFREDO

MAKES: *4* (1¼-CUP) SERVINGS · DIFFICULTY: *moderate*

If you don't have a spiralizer, don't worry. You can still make zucchini noodles right at home. Simply use an everyday vegetable peeler to scrape long, thin strands from the zucchini.

1 cup raw cashews, soaked for 4 hours and then drained

2 tablespoons nutritional yeast

2 teaspoons white miso paste

1½ cups Vegetable Broth (page 6) or water

½ ripe Hass avocado, peeled and pitted

1 tablespoon blended peeled lemon (see page 3)

4 to 6 medium zucchini, trimmed and spiralized or cut into long, thin, noodle-like strips

1 cup grape tomatoes, halved lengthwise

Ground black pepper or red pepper flakes

2 tablespoons minced fresh parsley or basil

Nutty Parm (page 4), to serve

Grind the drained cashews in a high-speed blender. Add the nutritional yeast, miso, and broth and blend until smooth. Add the avocado and lemon and blend until smooth, adding more broth, 1 tablespoon at a time, if the sauce is too thick. Set aside.

Steam the zucchini noodles over boiling water until tender, 2 to 4 minutes. Set aside.

In a large saucepan or deep skillet, warm the cashew sauce over low heat, stirring often. Add the zucchini noodles and tomatoes. Stir gently until the vegetables are heated through, about 5 minutes. If the sauce is too thick, add a little more broth to reach your desired consistency. When hot, serve at once, sprinkled with black pepper to taste, the parsley, and Nutty Parm.

SPIRALIZING

Traditional noodles are made of grains, but thanks to the spiralizer, you can make your own noodles out of vegetables. The spiralizer is an inexpensive tool that lets you turn fresh veggies into veggie-noodles.

Daily Dozen Foods

X OTHER FRUITS   X OTHER VEGETABLES   X NUTS AND SEEDS   X HERBS AND SPICES

PESTO CARROT NOODLES WITH WHITE BEANS & TOMATOES

MAKES: *4* (1½-CUP) SERVINGS · DIFFICULTY: *moderate*

Pesto is like a magic act: You take a green leafy vegetable (basil) and with just a little work, pesto presto! You turn it into a delicious sauce! The pesto in this recipe can also be enjoyed with your favorite whole-grain or bean pasta.

3 garlic cloves

1 teaspoon white miso paste

3 cups basil leaves

⅓ cup almonds or walnuts

2 tablespoons nutritional yeast

½ cup Vegetable Broth (page 6) or water

Ground black pepper

4 large carrots

1½ cups cooked or 1 15.5-ounce BPA-free can or Tetra Pak salt-free cannellini beans, drained and rinsed

1 cup grape or cherry tomatoes, halved lengthwise

Nutty Parm (page 4), to serve

In a food processor, combine the garlic and miso and process until the garlic is minced. Add the basil, nuts, and nutritional yeast and process until finely minced. Add the broth and black pepper to taste, and process until smooth, adding a little more broth if needed to achieve the desired texture for your pesto sauce. Set aside.

Cut the carrots into long, thin strips, using a spiralizer, mandoline, or vegetable peeler. Steam the carrot noodles until tender, 5 to 7 minutes. In a shallow bowl, combine the carrot noodles with the beans, tomatoes, and pesto sauce and toss gently to combine. Sprinkle with Nutty Parm and serve.

WALNUTS

Walnuts are probably the healthiest nuts, containing the most omega-3s and antioxidant power. They are my nuts of choice, and I often swap out other nuts in recipes for these to maximize the nutritional value of my meals.

Daily Dozen Foods

✗ BEANS   ✗ OTHER VEGETABLES   ✗ NUTS AND SEEDS   ✗ HERBS AND SPICES

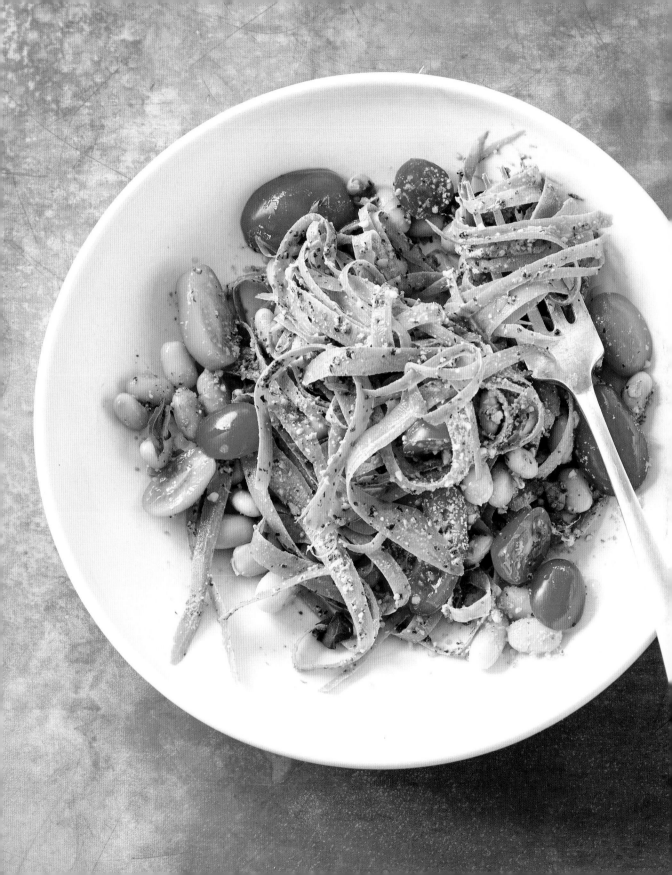

SPAGHETTI SQUASH ARRABIATA

MAKES: *4* (1¼-CUP) SERVINGS · DIFFICULTY: *easy*

Remember, as with most vegetables, the more colorful the squash, the more likely it's packed with antioxidants.

1 large (3-pound) spaghetti squash, cut in half

3 garlic cloves, minced

3 cups fresh, jarred, or Tetra Pak tomatoes, finely diced

2 tablespoons jarred tomato paste

1 teaspoon balsamic vinegar

1 teaspoon white miso paste

1 teaspoon dried basil

½ teaspoon red pepper flakes, or to taste

Savory Spice Blend (page 4)

¼ cup minced fresh parsley

Ground black pepper

Nutty Parm (page 4)

Preheat the oven to 350°F. Place the squash halves in a large baking dish, cut side up. Add 1 to 2 inches of water and tightly cover the dish. Bake until tender, 45 to 60 minutes.

While the squash is baking, make the sauce in a large skillet: Heat 2 tablespoons of water over medium heat. Add the garlic and cook for 1 minute to soften. Stir in all the remaining ingredients, except the Nutty Parm, and cook for 5 minutes longer. Keep warm.

When the squash is done baking, remove and discard its seeds. Use a fork to scrape the squash in strands and place in a large bowl. Add the sauce and toss gently to combine. Sprinkle with Nutty Parm and serve.

TIP: This arrabiata sauce also tastes great tossed with zucchini noodles or whole-grain pasta.

NUTS IN THE RAW

It's healthiest to eat nuts raw. When high-fat and high-protein foods are exposed to temperatures above 250°F, advanced glycation end products, or AGEs, are created. Appropriately acronymed, these so-called glycotoxins are thought to accelerate the aging process. The highest levels are found in broiled, roasted, fried, and barbequed meat, but AGEs can also occur when plant foods high in fat and protein, such as soy foods or nuts, are broiled or toasted.

Daily Dozen Foods

✗ OTHER VEGETABLES   ✗ NUTS AND SEEDS   ✗ HERBS AND SPICES

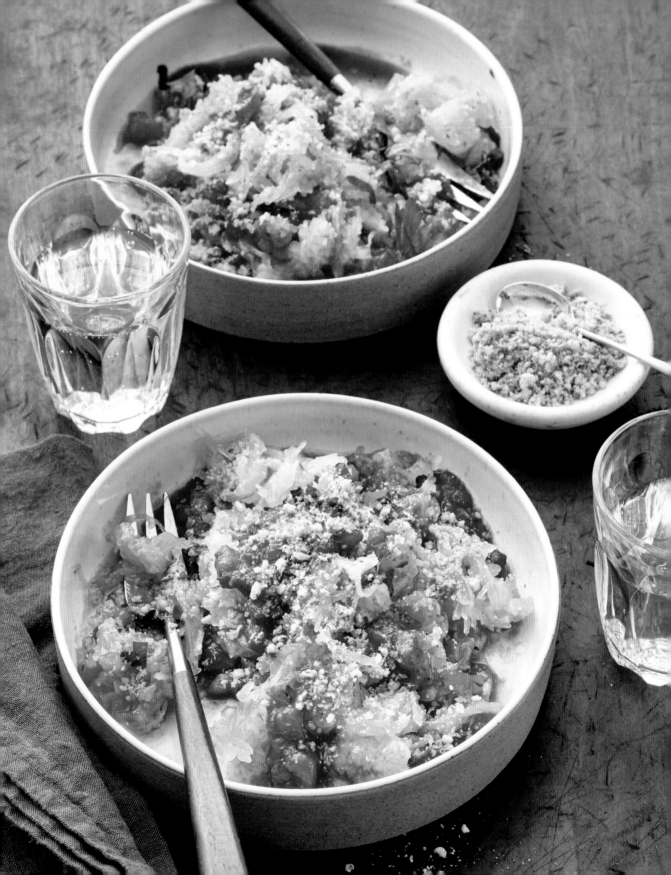

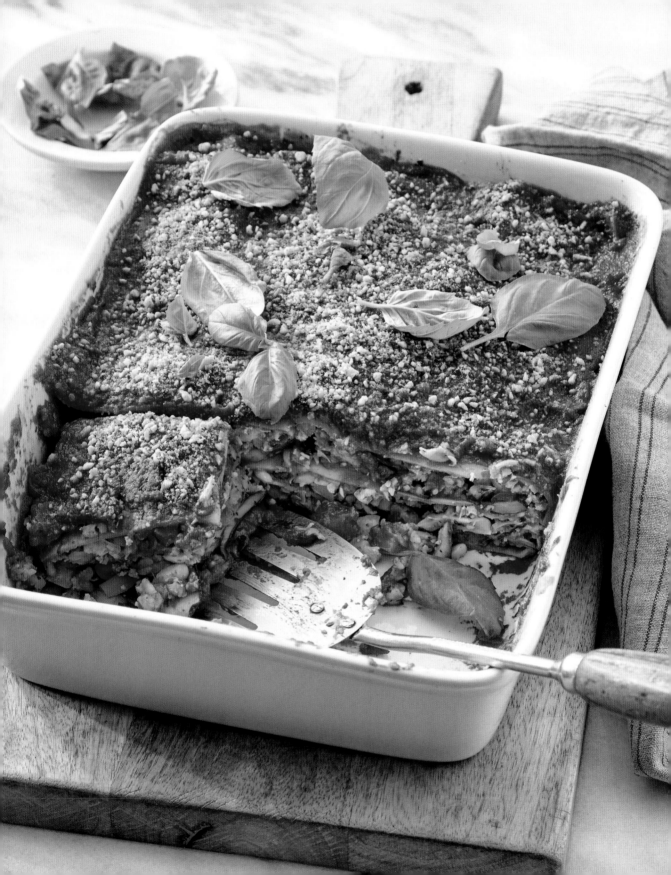

ROASTED VEGETABLE LASAGNA

MAKES: *6* (1¼-CUP) SERVINGS · DIFFICULTY: *moderate*

One of the wonderful things about lasagna is being able to truly make it your own. Not crazy about eggplant? Use sliced portobello mushrooms instead (as I do). Want to bulk it up? Add some crumbled steamed tempeh to the tomato sauce. And, as always, consider adding chopped greens to this—and everything else!

---

1 head cauliflower, cut vertically into ¼-inch slices

1 zucchini, cut into ⅛-inch slices

1 eggplant, cut into ⅛-inch slices

1 red bell pepper, seeded and chopped

12 100% whole-grain lasagna noodles

1½ cups cooked or 1 15.5-ounce BPA-free can or Tetra Pak cannellini beans, drained, rinsed, and mashed

¼ cup nutritional yeast

¼ cup minced fresh parsley

½ cup Almond Milk (page 2)

1 teaspoon blended peeled lemon (see page 3)

1 teaspoon white miso paste

1 teaspoon dried oregano

1 teaspoon dried basil

1 teaspoon garlic powder

1 teaspoon onion powder

¼ teaspoon red pepper flakes, or to taste

¼ teaspoon ground black pepper

3 cups jarred or homemade marinara sauce

¼ cup Nutty Parm (page 4)

Preheat the oven to 425°F. Line two large baking sheets with silicone mats or parchment paper. Arrange the cauliflower on one of the prepared baking sheets and the zucchini and eggplant on the other. Sprinkle the chopped bell pepper over the zucchini and eggplant. Place both pans of vegetables in the oven and roast until the veggies are tender, about 20 minutes, turning once about halfway through.

While the vegetables are roasting, cook the lasagna noodles according to the package directions. Drain and set aside.

Remove the roasted vegetables from the oven and set aside to cool. Lower the oven temperature to 350°F.

Transfer the roasted cauliflower to a food processor and pulse until it is finely chopped. Place the cauliflower in a large bowl and add the remaining ingredients, except the marinara sauce and Nutty Parm. Mix well.

To assemble, spread a layer of marinara sauce on the bottom of a 9 × 13-inch baking dish. Top the sauce with a layer of noodles. Cover the noodles with half of the roasted vegetables, topped with half of the cauliflower mixture. Add another layer of noodles, topped with more sauce. Once again cover the noodles with roasted vegetables, and then the cauliflower mixture. Repeat this layering process, ending with a layer of noodles topped with sauce. Sprinkle Nutty Parm on top. Cover and bake for 30 to 40 minutes, or until hot and bubbling. Remove from the oven and let stand for 10 minutes before cutting and serving.

Daily Dozen Foods

✗ BEANS   ✗ OTHER VEGETABLES   ✗ NUTS AND SEEDS   ✗ HERBS AND SPICES   ✗ WHOLE GRAINS

STUFFED PORTOBELLOS WITH HERBED MUSHROOM GRAVY

MAKES: *4* SERVINGS · DIFFICULTY: *easy*

If I had been preparing a Daily *Baker*'s Dozen, mushrooms would probably have made my list. Though the evidence isn't quite as strong, there's a lot of interesting new research that touts the benefits mushrooms offer, especially on improving immune function. If I don't have fresh mushrooms on hand, then dried will do. I cook them in soups, add them to pasta sauces, or make them the star player, as in this dish.

4 large portobello mushroom caps, stems removed

2 scallions, coarsely chopped

2 garlic cloves, minced

3 cups spinach leaves, loosely packed

1½ cups cooked or 1 15.5-ounce BPA-free can or Tetra Pak salt-free chickpeas, drained and rinsed

2 tablespoons tahini

2 tablespoons nutritional yeast

2 tablespoons white miso paste

1 teaspoon blended peeled lemon (see page 3)

½ teaspoon onion powder

½ teaspoon smoked paprika

Ground black pepper

½ cup 100% whole-grain bread crumbs

2 tablespoons ground flaxseeds

2 shallots, finely minced

2 cups chopped, assorted fresh mushrooms

1½ cups Vegetable Broth (page 6)

1 teaspoon dried thyme

½ teaspoon dried sage

2 tablespoons chopped fresh parsley

Preheat the oven to 400°F. Arrange the mushroom caps, stem side down, in a large baking dish with ¼ cup of water and bake for 10 minutes to soften.

While the mushrooms are baking, make the stuffing: In a food processor, combine the scallions, garlic, spinach, and chickpeas and process until finely minced. Add the tahini, nutritional yeast, 1 tablespoon of the miso, and the lemon, onion powder, paprika, and black pepper to taste. Pulse to combine. Add the bread crumbs and flaxseeds and pulse once again to combine while retaining some texture in the chickpeas. Flip over the baked mushrooms and spoon the stuffing mixture into the mushroom caps, gently pressing the stuffing into each cap. Bake for about 20 minutes, or until the mushrooms are tender and the stuffing is hot.

While the stuffed mushrooms are baking, make the gravy: Heat 2 tablespoons of water in a skillet over medium heat. Add the shallot and cook until soft, about 3 minutes. Add the chopped, assorted mushrooms and cook for 2 to 3 minutes to soften. Stir in the broth, remaining tablespoon of miso, thyme, sage, and black pepper to taste. Bring to a boil, then reduce the heat to low and simmer for 5 minutes. Transfer the mixture to a blender or food processor and blend until smooth.

Serve the stuffed mushrooms hot with the gravy spooned over top and sprinkled with parsley.

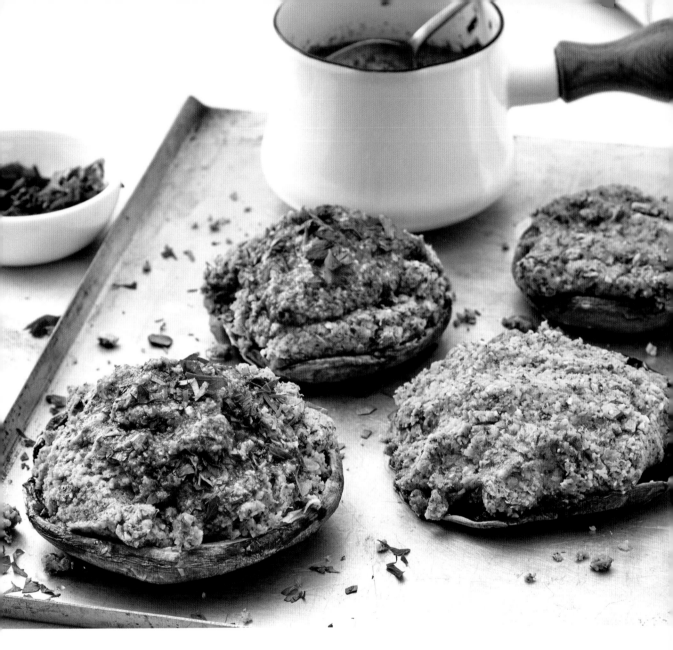

TIP: The gravy is also delicious as a topping for the Black Bean Burgers (page 88) and the Red Quinoa Loaf (page 156).

Daily Dozen Foods

✗ BEANS   ✗ GREENS   ✗ OTHER VEGETABLES   ✗ FLAXSEEDS   ✗ NUTS AND SEEDS   ✗ HERBS AND SPICES

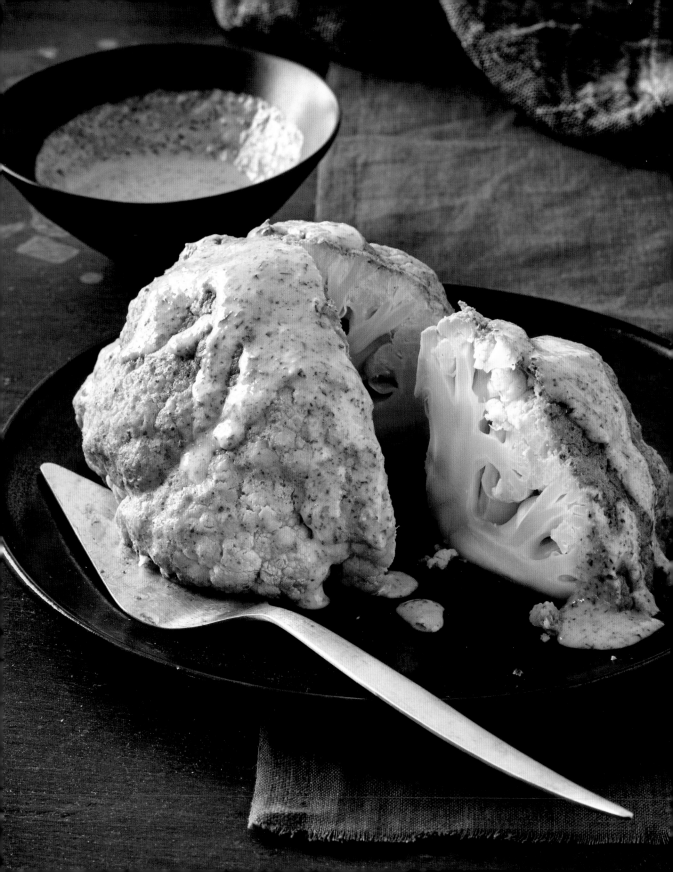

WHOLE ROASTED CAULIFLOWER WITH LEMON TAHINI SAUCE

MAKES: *4* (1-CUP) SERVINGS · DIFFICULTY: *easy*

Cauliflower is another nutritious plant that can be served many ways—roasted, boiled, sautéed, broiled, steamed, or raw. The whole cauliflower in this dish makes a great-looking centerpiece on the dinner table.

---

3 garlic cloves, crushed

2 teaspoons white miso paste

1 tablespoon tahini

1½ tablespoons blended peeled lemon (see page 3)

2 tablespoons nutritional yeast

½ teaspoon salt-free stone-ground mustard

1 ¼-inch piece fresh turmeric, grated (or ¼ teaspoon ground)

Savory Spice Blend (page 4)

1 head cauliflower, leaves and tough stem removed

3 tablespoons chopped fresh parsley

Ground black pepper

In a food processor or blender, combine the garlic and miso and process until the garlic is finely minced. Add ½ cup of water and the tahini, lemon, nutritional yeast, mustard, turmeric, and Savory Spice Blend to taste and blend the sauce until smooth. Set aside.

Bring water to boil in a pot large enough for the cauliflower to be immersed fully. Place the cauliflower carefully in the boiling water. Cover and cook until blanched, about 8 minutes.

Preheat the oven to 400°F.

Transfer the cauliflower to a shallow baking dish, stem side down, and add ½ inch of water. Spoon about half of the sauce on top of the cauliflower and use your fingers to rub the sauce onto the cauliflower. Roast until the cauliflower is tender, about 40 minutes. Stir the parsley and black pepper to taste into the remaining sauce and adjust the seasonings, if needed. Heat the remaining sauce in a small saucepan or microwave. When the cauliflower is ready, transfer it to a platter and top with the remaining sauce. Serve hot.

CAULIFLOWER

If you added only one thing to your diet, consider cruciferous vegetables, such as cauliflower. Less than a single serving a day of cauliflower, broccoli, Brussels sprouts, cabbage, or kale may cut the risk of certain cancers progressing by more than half.[120]

Daily Dozen Foods

X CRUCIFEROUS VEGETABLES   X NUTS AND SEEDS   X HERBS AND SPICES

VEGETABLE STACKS WITH TOMATO-RED PEPPER COULIS

MAKES: *4* SERVINGS · DIFFICULTY: *moderate*

This dish takes a little extra time to assemble, but the bit of effort is so very worth it. It's actually a quite simple dish to make and looks very fancy when plated. Perfect for when you want to impress your dining companion!

---

1 large eggplant, trimmed and cut into 4 round slices about ½-inch thick

1 large red onion, cut into 4 slices about ½-inch thick

1 large orange or yellow bell pepper, sides cut vertically to make 4 square pieces

4 large portobello mushroom caps, gills removed

1 or 2 large ripe tomatoes, cut into 4 slices about ½-inch thick

3 tablespoons minced red onion

2 plum tomatoes, chopped

2 roasted red bell peppers (see page 9, or store-bought)

1 teaspoon white miso paste

1 teaspoon dried basil

½ teaspoon dried thyme

1 ¼-inch piece fresh turmeric, grated (or ¼ teaspoon ground)

Ground black pepper

Fresh parsley for garnish

Preheat the oven to 425°F.

Line two large baking sheets with silicone mats or parchment paper. Arrange the eggplant slices in a single layer on one of the prepared baking sheets. Bake the eggplant until soft, turning once, about 15 minutes. Remove the baking sheet from the oven and set aside to cool; then remove the eggplant from the pan. Meanwhile, on the second prepared baking sheet, arrange the onion slices in a single layer and bake for 7 to 8 minutes. Turn over the onion slices, place the bell pepper pieces on the same baking sheet as the onion, and roast until the vegetables are tender, about 15 minutes longer. Set aside to cool. Arrange the mushroom caps, gill side up, on the baking sheet from which the eggplant has been removed. Roast until softened, about 10 minutes. Set aside to cool for a few minutes.

Lower the oven temperature to 350°F. Assemble the roasted vegetables in stacks: To begin, leave the four mushroom caps, gill side up, on their baking sheet. Top each cap with a slice of eggplant, followed by a slice of onion, then a bell pepper slice, topped with a slice of tomato. Cover the baking sheet and bake until the vegetables are hot, about 20 minutes.

While the vegetables are cooking, make the sauce: In a skillet, heat 3 tablespoons of water over medium heat and add the minced onion. Cover and cook for 4 minutes, or until soft. Stir in the plum tomatoes, roasted bell peppers, miso, basil, thyme, turmeric, and black pepper to taste. Cover and cook until the vegetables are very soft, about 5 minutes longer. Transfer to a food processor and purée the sauce until smooth. Keep warm over low heat until ready to use.

Daily Dozen Foods

X OTHER VEGETABLES   X HERBS AND SPICES

When the stacks are ready, use a metal spatula to carefully remove them from the baking dish. Place one stack in the center of each of four dinner plates. Top and surround each stack with the sauce and parsley garnish, and serve hot.

TIP: For a more attractive dish, cut the stackable vegetables slices so they are approximately the same size. Reserve the remaining pieces of the vegetables for another use.

CAULIFLOWER STEAKS WITH CHERMOULA SAUCE

MAKES: *4* (1½-CUP) SERVINGS · DIFFICULTY: *easy*

Chermoula is a sauce found in Northern African cuisine, most often made of a mixture of herbs, oil, lemon juice, pickled lemons, garlic, cumin, and salt. It may also include onion, cilantro, ground chili peppers, black pepper, or saffron. It's one of the most dramatic flavors I've tasted and elevates this meaty steak to another level. Serve this dish over quinoa or brown, red, or black rice for a spectacular meal.

1 head cauliflower, trimmed, cored, and cut into ½-inch-thick slices

3 garlic cloves, crushed

¾ cup coarsely chopped fresh parsley

¾ cup coarsely chopped fresh cilantro

1 ¼-inch piece fresh turmeric, grated (or ¼ teaspoon ground)

1 teaspoon white miso paste

½ teaspoon ground coriander

½ teaspoon ground cumin

½ teaspoon smoked paprika

¼ teaspoon ground ginger

¼ teaspoon cayenne pepper

1 tablespoon blended peeled lemon (see page 3)

Preheat the oven to 425°F.

Arrange the cauliflower slices on a large baking sheet lined with a silicone mat or parchment paper. Roast until just tender, about 15 minutes, turning once halfway through.

In a food processor, combine the garlic, parsley, cilantro, and turmeric and process until finely minced. Add the miso, coriander, cumin, paprika, ginger, cayenne, lemon, and ¼ cup of water. Process until the sauce is smooth. Set aside.

Remove the roasted cauliflower from the oven and use a metal spatula to transfer it to a shallow serving platter. Serve hot, topped with the sauce.

Daily Dozen Foods

✗ CRUCIFEROUS VEGETABLES   ✗ HERBS AND SPICES

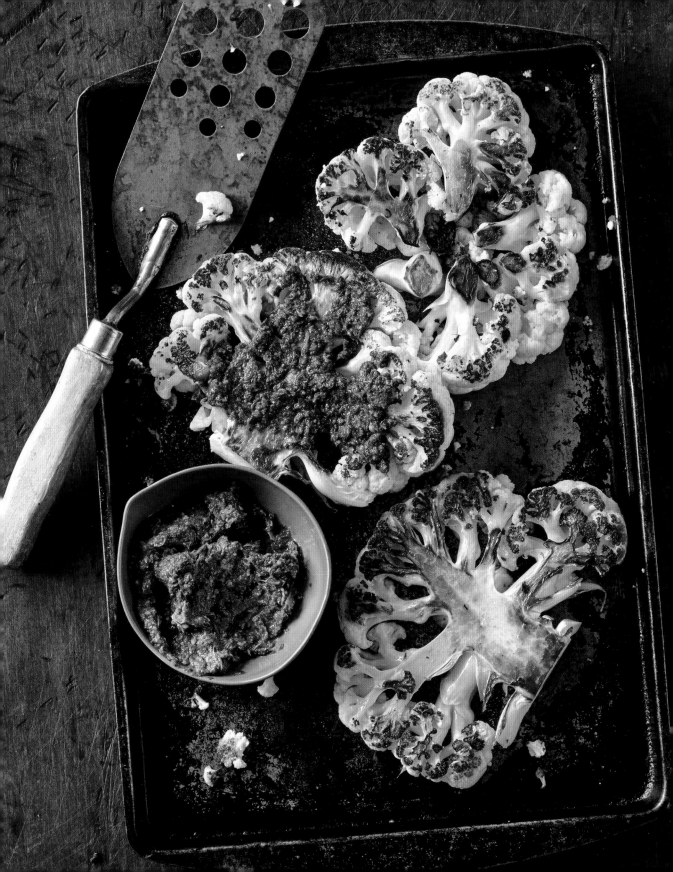

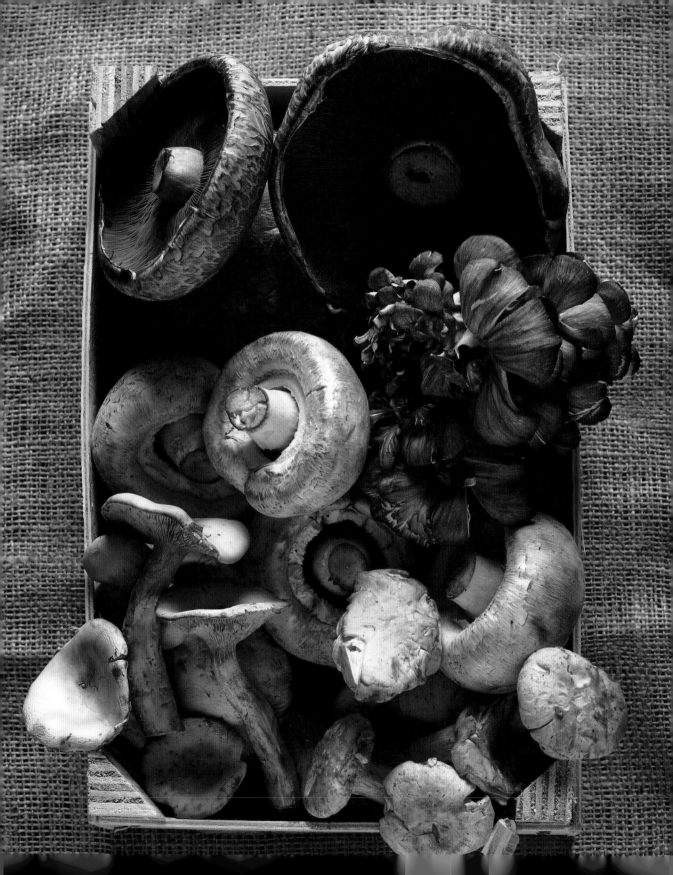

PORTOBELLOS & GREENS ON TOAST

MAKES: *4* SERVINGS (1 SLICE BREAD + 1 CUP PORTOBELLOS & GREENS PER SERVING) · DIFFICULTY: *easy*

As much as I love mushrooms, they are seldom a main dish for me. Portobellos are the exception because they're so hearty and satisfying. This open-faced, knife-and-fork sandwich makes a quick and easy lunch or dinner entrée.

8 to 12 ounces portobello mushroom caps, thinly sliced

3 scallions, minced

6 cups chopped spinach or chard

1 teaspoon dried thyme

½ teaspoon smoked paprika

¼ teaspoon ground black pepper

2 tablespoons Umami Sauce (page 5)

½ teaspoon salt-free stone-ground mustard

⅓ cup Almond Milk (page 2)

4 slices 100% whole-grain bread

2 tablespoons chopped fresh parsley

Heat 2 tablespoons of water in a large skillet over medium-high heat. Add the portobellos and stir-fry until softened. Add the scallions and spinach and cook, stirring, for 1 to 2 minutes to wilt the greens. Add the thyme, paprika, black pepper, Umami Sauce, mustard, and Almond Milk, stirring to blend well, and cook for 1 to 2 minutes longer to thicken slightly. Keep warm while you toast the bread. Once the bread is toasted, cut the slices in half and arrange them on plates. Top with the portobellos and greens and sprinkle with parsley. Serve warm.

VARIATIONS: Add 1 cup of cooked beans. Serve over brown, black, or red rice or another whole grain instead of toast. If you prefer, try shiitakes instead of portobellos. Likewise, you can use kale or tatsoi instead of spinach or chard.

MUSHROOMS

Mushrooms may be able to boost immune function. An Australian study found that people eating a cup of cooked white button mushrooms every day can elevate their saliva IgA levels—antibodies that neutralize and prevent viruses from penetrating into the body—by as much as 50 percent.[123] This appears to translate into fewer viral infections.[124]

Daily Dozen Foods

✗ GREENS   ✗ OTHER VEGETABLES   ✗ HERBS AND SPICES   ✗ WHOLE GRAINS

EIGHT

BEAN CUISINE

This chapter features beans every which way, from the more exotic Chickpea & Vegetable Tagine, Bean Patties with Harissa, and Yellow Split Pea Dal with Watercress to Daily Dozen–inspired takes on down-home favorites, such as Smoky Black-Eyed Peas & Collards and Lentil Shepherd's Pie. Recipes using tempeh and Soy Curls are also featured, and I hope you love the Braised Tempeh & Bok Choy with Spicy Ginger Sauce and Louisiana-Style Soy Curls as much as I do.

CHICKPEA & VEGETABLE TAGINE

SMOKY BLACK-EYED PEAS & COLLARDS

BRAISED TEMPEH & BOK CHOY
WITH SPICY GINGER SAUCE

CHICKPEA & CAULIFLOWER CURRY

LENTIL SHEPHERD'S PIE

YELLOW SPLIT PEA DAL WITH WATERCRESS

LOUISIANA-STYLE SOY CURLS

BEAN PATTIES WITH HARISSA

CHICKPEA & VEGETABLE TAGINE

MAKES: *4* (1¼-CUP) SERVINGS · DIFFICULTY: *easy*

Lots of spices combine with lots of veggies for a great-tasting dish that is especially good served over quinoa or brown, red, or black rice. Common to North African cuisine, *tagine* refers both to the earthenware pot in which the food is cooked as well as the food itself.

1 red onion, chopped

1 carrot, chopped

1 green bell pepper, seeded and chopped

1 garlic clove, minced

1½ teaspoons minced fresh ginger

2 tablespoons jarred tomato paste

¼ teaspoon ground cinnamon

½ teaspoon ground cumin

½ teaspoon smoked paprika

1 ¼-inch piece fresh turmeric, grated (or ¼ teaspoon ground)

⅛ to ¼ teaspoon cayenne pepper, or to taste

2 cups Vegetable Broth (page 6)

1 cup green beans, cut into 1-inch pieces

2 cups diced mushrooms

1½ cups cooked or 1 15.5-ounce BPA-free can or Tetra Pak salt-free chickpeas, drained and rinsed

2 tablespoons minced fresh cilantro or parsley

2 teaspoons blended peeled lemon (see page 3)

1 tablespoon raisins or minced dried apricot

Heat ¼ cup of water in a large saucepan over medium heat. Add the onion, carrot, and bell pepper. Cover and cook for 5 minutes. Stir in the garlic, ginger, tomato paste, cinnamon, cumin, paprika, turmeric, and cayenne. Add the broth, green beans, mushrooms, and chickpeas and bring to a boil. Reduce the heat to low, cover, and simmer until the vegetables are tender, about 20 minutes. Stir in the cilantro, lemon, and raisins and cook 5 minutes longer. Taste to adjust the seasonings, and serve hot.

Daily Dozen Foods

𝑋 BEANS   𝑋 OTHER FRUITS   𝑋 OTHER VEGETABLES   𝑋 HERBS AND SPICES

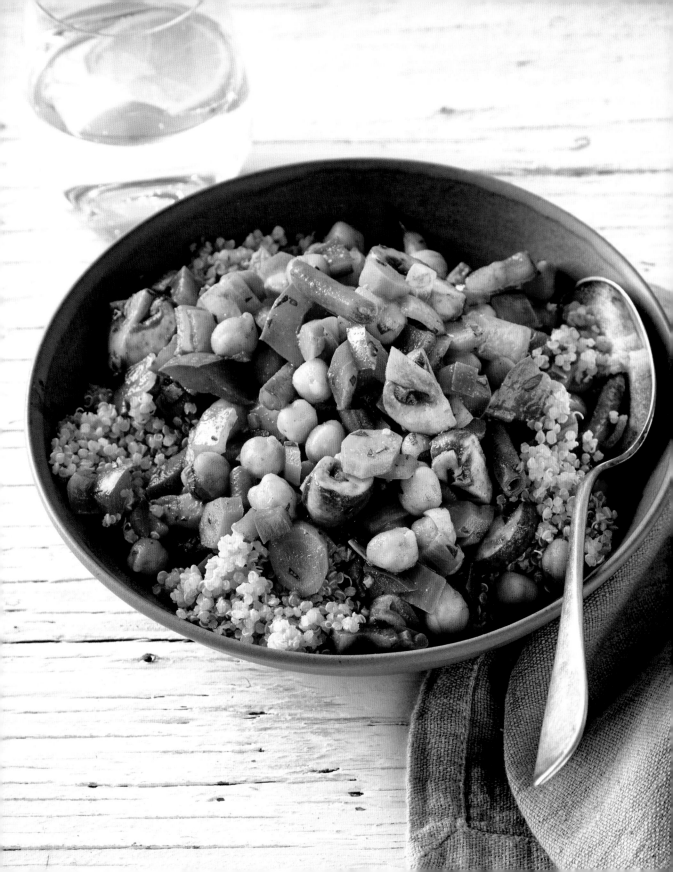

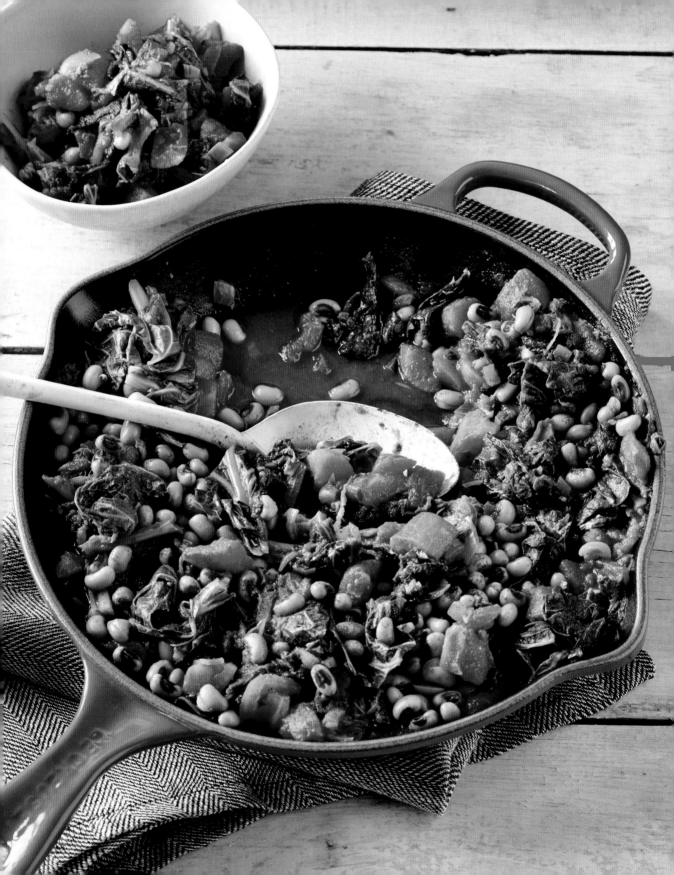

SMOKY BLACK-EYED PEAS & COLLARDS

MAKES: *4* (1¼-CUP) SERVINGS · DIFFICULTY: *easy*

This Southern classic is a delicious way to enjoy your greens. If fresh collards are unavailable, substitute frozen collards or another dark green leafy vegetable, such as kale. I can't get enough of this dish, especially when it's over quinoa or brown, black, or red rice.

1½ pounds fresh collard greens, well washed, tough stems removed

1 small red onion, chopped

1 garlic clove, minced

1 teaspoon smoked paprika

1 ¼-inch piece fresh turmeric, grated (or ¼ teaspoon ground)

Savory Spice Blend (page 4)

1 teaspoon white miso paste

1 14.5-ounce BPA-free can or Tetra Pak salt-free diced tomatoes, drained

1½ cups cooked or 1 15.5-ounce BPA-free can or Tetra Pak salt-free black-eyed peas, drained and rinsed

Healthy Hot Sauce (page 8)

Cook the collard greens in a pot of boiling water until tender, about 20 minutes. Drain well, reserving ¼ cup of the cooking water; then coarsely chop the collards and set aside. Heat the reserved cooking water in a large skillet over medium heat. Add the onion, garlic, paprika, turmeric, and Savory Spice Blend to taste. Cover and cook until the onions are soft, about 4 minutes. Stir in the miso, tomatoes, black-eyed peas, collards, and Healthy Hot Sauce to taste. Simmer to heat through and combine the flavors, about 10 minutes. Serve hot.

Daily Dozen Foods

X BEANS   X GREENS   X OTHER VEGETABLES   X HERBS AND SPICES

BRAISED TEMPEH & BOK CHOY WITH SPICY GINGER SAUCE

MAKES: *4* (2-CUP) SERVINGS · DIFFICULTY: *moderate*

Although tofu is highly nutritious, I prefer tempeh as it is a *whole* soy food with fewer nutrients removed. I love it in this dish, but you can also modify this recipe with ease by skipping the tempeh and adding more bok choy or other veggies with a different bean.

16 ounces tempeh, cut into ½-inch dice

1 cup Vegetable Broth (page 6) or water

1 medium red onion, chopped

3 to 4 small heads baby bok choy, trimmed and halved lengthwise, or 5 cups coarsely chopped bok choy

3 garlic cloves, minced

2 tablespoons grated fresh ginger

2 tablespoons white miso paste

1 tablespoon rice vinegar

2 tablespoons Umami Sauce (page 5)

½ teaspoon red pepper flakes, or to taste

1 teaspoon date sugar

½ red bell pepper, minced

1 cup chopped mushrooms

4 scallions, chopped

Steam the tempeh in a steamer basket over boiling water for 15 minutes. Uncover and set aside.

Heat ¼ cup of the broth in a large skillet or wok over medium-high heat. Add the onion and bok choy, and cook, stirring until tender, about 5 minutes. Remove from the skillet and set aside.

Heat the remaining ¾ cup of broth in the same skillet over medium heat. Stir in the garlic, ginger, miso, vinegar, Umami Sauce, red pepper flakes, and date sugar. Add the bell pepper, mushrooms, scallions, and steamed tempeh and stir to combine. Lower the heat to a simmer and cook for 5 minutes longer, stirring occasionally. Add the onion and bok choy, and cook for about 3 minutes longer to heat through. Serve hot.

GINGER

A double-blind, randomized, controlled clinical trial compared the efficacy of ginger for the treatment of migraine headaches to sumatriptan (Imitrex), one of the top-selling drugs in the world. A pinch of powdered ginger worked just as well and just as fast as the drug[125] (and costs less than a penny). Ginger can also help with menstrual cramps, which plague up to 90 percent of younger women. Just ⅛ teaspoon of ginger powder three times a day started a few days before one's period was found to drop pain from an 8 to a 6 on a scale of 1 to 10, and down further to a 3 in the following month.[126]

Daily Dozen Foods

✗ BEANS   ✗ CRUCIFEROUS VEGETABLES   ✗ OTHER VEGETABLES   ✗ HERBS AND SPICES

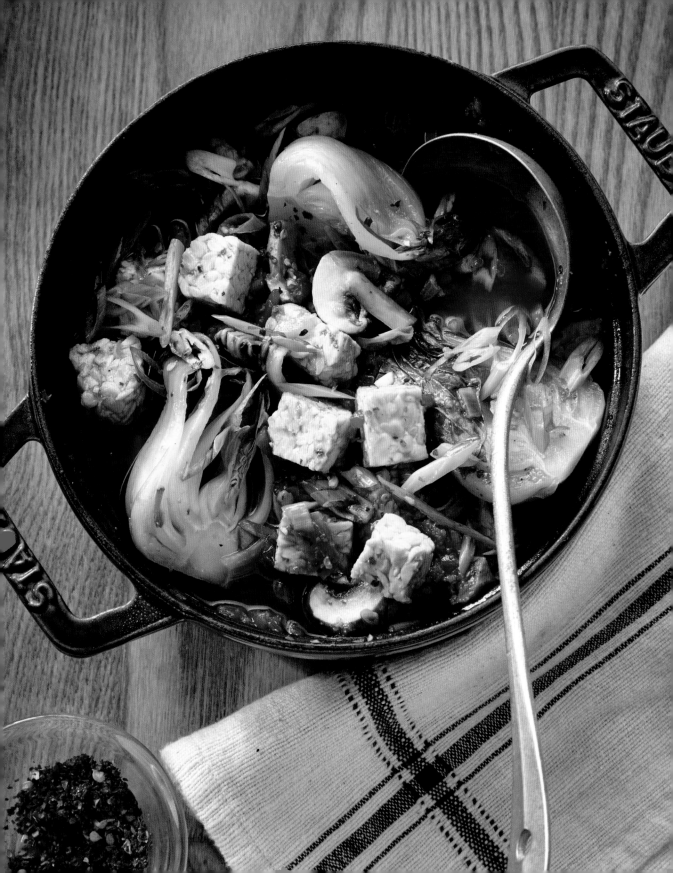

CHICKPEA & CAULIFLOWER CURRY

MAKES: *4* (2-CUP) SERVINGS · DIFFICULTY: *easy*

This curry marries legumes and cruciferous vegetables, two of the superstar plant families, in a match made in heaven. If you aren't in the mood for green beans, substitute green peas or edamame. Serve over cooked brown rice.

1 cup Vegetable Broth (page 6)

1 red onion, chopped

2 garlic cloves, chopped

1 jalapeño pepper, seeded and minced (optional)

1½ tablespoons curry powder

1 head cauliflower, trimmed and cut into small florets

8 ounces green beans, trimmed and cut into 1-inch pieces

1 14.5-ounce BPA-free can or Tetra Pak salt-free diced tomatoes, undrained

2 roasted red bell peppers (see page 9, or store-bought), chopped

1 cup Almond Milk (page 2)

3 tablespoons nutritional yeast

½ teaspoon smoked paprika

1½ cups cooked or 1 15.5-ounce BPA-free can or Tetra Pak salt-free chickpeas, drained and rinsed

Cooked brown rice, to serve

In a large pot, heat the broth to a boil over medium-high heat. Add the onion and garlic, cover, and cook until tender, about 3 minutes. Stir in the jalapeño (if using) and curry powder; then add the cauliflower, green beans, tomatoes, and roasted bell peppers. Cover and bring to a boil. Reduce the heat to low and simmer until the vegetables are tender, about 20 minutes.

When the veggies are tender, use an immersion blender to break up some of the vegetables. Alternatively, remove up to 2 cups of the solids and liquids from the pot, purée in a blender or food processor, and then return the mixture to the pot. Stir in the Almond Milk, nutritional yeast, smoked paprika, and chickpeas, and cook 5 to 10 minutes longer to heat through and blend the flavors. Serve over a bed of cooked brown rice.

Daily Dozen Foods

✗ BEANS   ✗ CRUCIFEROUS VEGETABLES   ✗ OTHER VEGETABLES   ✗ HERBS AND SPICES   ✗ WHOLE GRAINS

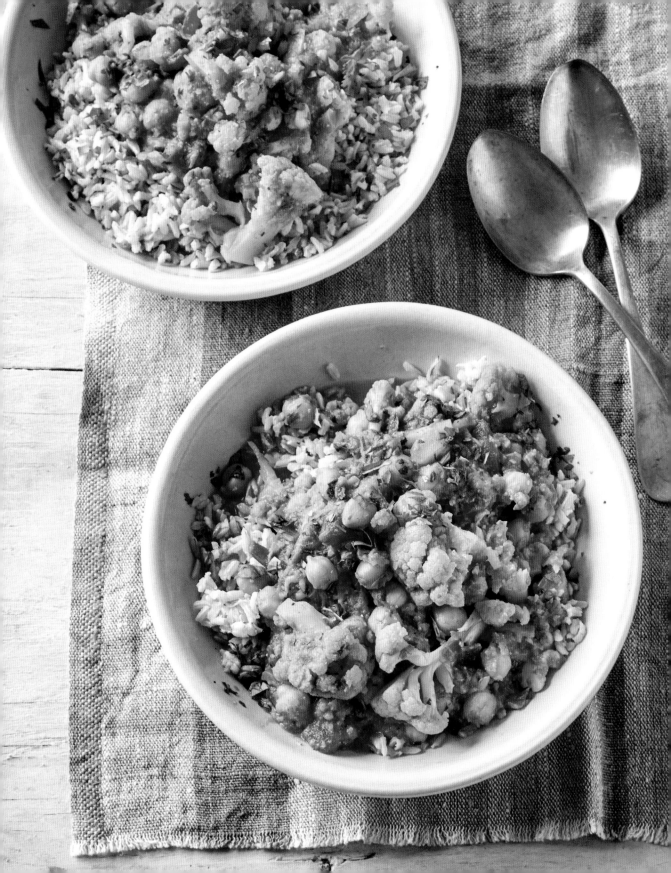

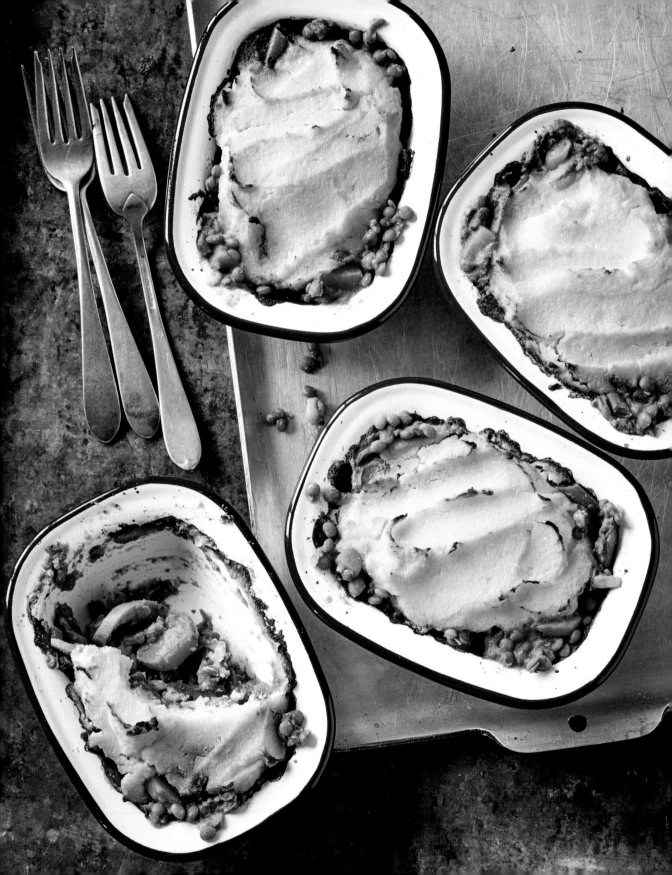

LENTIL SHEPHERD'S PIE

MAKES: *4* SERVINGS · DIFFICULTY: *moderate*

Lentils can be transformed into a delicious, nutritious soup you can make in a snap. If you're feeling a little more ambitious, you can make a meal like this wonderful savory pie.

1 small red onion, chopped

1 carrot, chopped

6 ounces green beans, trimmed and cut into ½-inch pieces

1 zucchini or yellow (summer) squash, chopped

1 cup Vegetable Broth (page 6)

8 ounces mushrooms, chopped

1 tablespoon plus 1 teaspoon white miso paste

2 tablespoons Umami Sauce (page 5)

1 teaspoon minced fresh thyme or ½ teaspoon dried

3 tablespoons nutritional yeast

Ground black pepper

2 cups cooked lentils

Cauliflower Mash (page 175)

Steam the onion, carrot, and green beans in a steamer basket over boiling water for 5 minutes. Add the zucchini and steam for 3 minutes longer, or until the vegetables are tender. Drain and set aside in a shallow baking dish.

Heat the broth in a saucepan over medium heat. Add the mushrooms, miso, Umami Sauce, thyme, 2 tablespoons of the nutritional yeast, and black pepper to taste. Cook, stirring, for 5 minutes, or until the mushrooms are soft. Transfer to a blender or food processor. Add ½ cup of the cooked lentils and blend until smooth. Add up to ½ cup of additional broth to make the gravy smoother, as desired. Combine the gravy with the remaining 1½ cups of lentils, add to the steamed vegetables, and stir. Set aside.

Preheat the oven to 375°F. Stir the remaining 1 tablespoon of nutritional yeast into the Cauliflower Mash; then spoon it on top of the lentils and vegetables, smoothing to cover the surface. Bake until hot, 30 to 40 minutes.

TIP: To save some time, you can substitute about 3 cups of frozen mixed vegetables for the carrot, green beans, and zucchini. Simply steam them, and then proceed with the recipe.

Daily Dozen Foods

X BEANS   X CRUCIFEROUS VEGETABLES   X OTHER VEGETABLES   X HERBS AND SPICES

YELLOW SPLIT PEA DAL WITH WATERCRESS

MAKES: *4* (1¼-CUP) SERVINGS · DIFFICULTY: *easy*

My favorite way of preparing split peas is to make a warm and comforting soup. (It's a classic for a reason.) I also throw split peas in the rice cooker, the way I prepare lentils. The following is yet another way to add these nutritious little gems into your daily diet. Remember: In my ideal world, we're all enjoying legumes (beans, chickpeas, split peas, or lentils) with every meal.

If you prefer, use any type of lentil instead of the yellow split peas in this recipe. Don't have watercress? Use spinach or arugula instead. Serve this gorgeous dal over brown, black, or red rice. *Dal*, by the way, is the Indian word for "split pea," or a dish made with them.

1½ cups dried yellow split peas, picked through and rinsed

3 cups Vegetable Broth (page 6) or water

3 cups coarsely chopped watercress or spinach

1 14.5-ounce BPA-free can or Tetra Pak salt-free diced petite tomatoes, drained

¼ cup chopped fresh cilantro

2 garlic cloves, minced

1 tablespoon finely chopped fresh ginger

1 small hot green chili, seeded and minced

2 tablespoons nutritional yeast

1 teaspoon white miso paste

1 teaspoon ground cumin

½ teaspoon ground coriander

1 ¼-inch piece fresh turmeric, grated (or ¼ teaspoon ground)

2 teaspoons blended peeled lemon (see page 3)

Cover the split peas with boiling water and soak for 1 hour. Drain, then transfer to a saucepan with the broth and bring to a boil. Lower the heat to a simmer and cook until the split peas are tender, 45 to 60 minutes, adding a little more broth, if needed.

When the split peas are soft, add the watercress, tomatoes, and cilantro, stirring to wilt the watercress. Keep warm over very low heat.

Heat 2 tablespoons of water in a small skillet over medium heat. Add the garlic, ginger, and chili. Cook until softened, about 1 minute. Remove from the heat and add the nutritional yeast, miso, cumin, coriander, turmeric, and lemon, stirring to mix well. Add the spice mixture to the split pea dal, stirring to combine. Serve hot.

Daily Dozen Foods

✗ BEANS   ✗ GREENS   ✗ OTHER VEGETABLES   ✗ HERBS AND SPICES

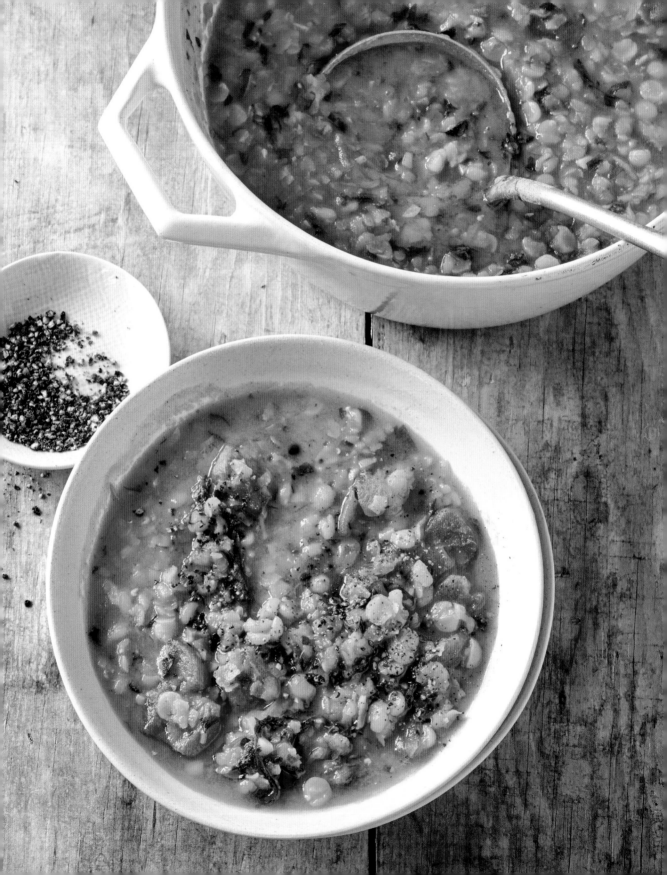

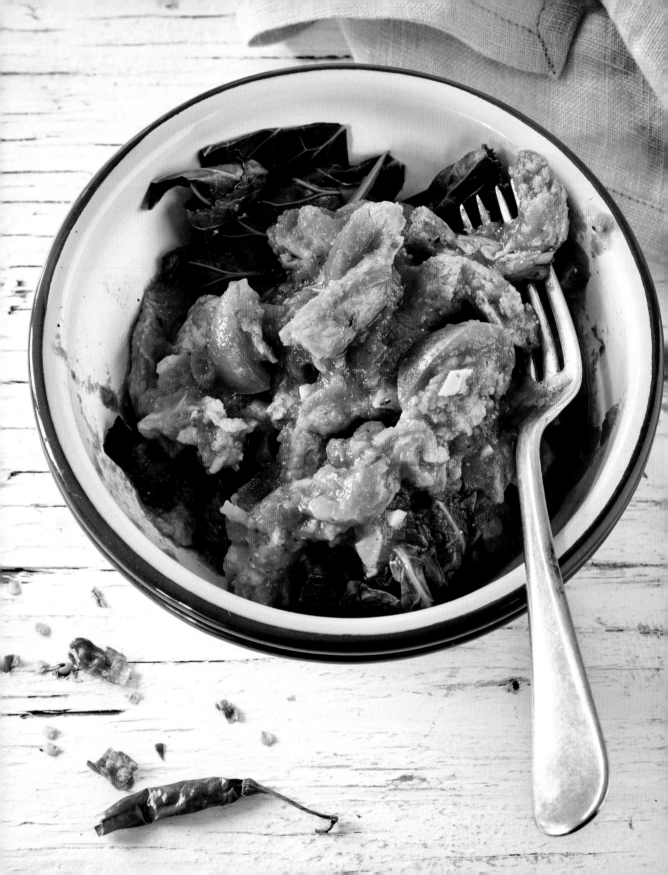

LOUISIANA-STYLE SOY CURLS

MAKES: *4* (1¼-CUP) SERVINGS · DIFFICULTY: *easy*

Soy Curls are a shelf-stable meat substitute containing a single ingredient—whole soybeans—that are available at natural food stores or online. If you prefer, you can substitute 8 ounces of steamed, diced tempeh or 1½ cups of cooked or canned dark red kidney beans.
This Creole-inspired dish is best served on a bed of cooked greens or whole grains.

1 cup Soy Curls

1¼ cups Vegetable Broth (page 6) or water

1 tablespoon salt-free Creole seasoning blend

2 tablespoons jarred tomato paste

2 teaspoons white miso paste

1 large red onion, chopped

1 large green bell pepper, seeded and chopped

2 celery ribs, chopped

3 garlic cloves, chopped

1 14.5-ounce BPA-free can or Tetra Pak salt-free diced tomatoes, drained

2 bay leaves

1 teaspoon dried thyme

½ teaspoon dried basil

Savory Spice Blend (page 4)

Ground black pepper

Healthy Hot Sauce (page 8)

Place the Soy Curls in a large saucepan with the broth and Creole seasoning. Bring to a boil. Cover and simmer for 5 minutes. Stir in the tomato paste, miso, onion, bell pepper, celery, and garlic. Cover and cook until the vegetables are softened, about 10 minutes. Stir in the tomatoes, bay leaves, thyme, basil, Savory Spice Blend, and black pepper to taste and cook, uncovered, for about 15 minutes to blend the flavors and reduce the liquid. Remove the bay leaves before serving with Healthy Hot Sauce.

Daily Dozen Foods

X BEANS   X OTHER VEGETABLES   X HERBS AND SPICES

BEAN PATTIES WITH HARISSA

MAKES: *4* SERVINGS · DIFFICULTY: *easy*

There are dozens of ways to make delicious patties. One reason I love this recipe so much is that the patties are heartier and nuttier than most, which make for an even better meal. Rather than in a bun, serve this dish on a bed of cooked greens.

1 tablespoon ground flaxseeds

2 teaspoons blended peeled lemon (see page 3)

½ cup old-fashioned rolled oats

1½ cups cooked or 1 15.5-ounce BPA-free can or Tetra Pak salt-free kidney beans or black beans, drained and rinsed

½ cup chopped walnuts

½ cup chopped onion

2 garlic cloves

1 ¼-inch piece fresh turmeric, grated (or ¼ teaspoon ground)

2 tablespoons tahini

2 tablespoons nutritional yeast

1 tablespoon white miso paste

½ teaspoon smoked paprika

2 tablespoons minced fresh parsley

Harissa (page 9)

In a small bowl, combine the flaxseeds and lemon, stirring until well blended. Set aside. Grind the oats into a coarse flour in a food processor. Add the beans, walnuts, onion, garlic, and turmeric and process until well combined. Add the tahini, nutritional yeast, miso, paprika, parsley, and flaxseed mixture. Pulse until well combined. Shape into four patties. (They will be sticky.) Place the patties on a baking sheet lined with a silicone mat or parchment paper and refrigerate for 30 minutes. Preheat the oven to 350°F. Bake the patties for 30 minutes; then flip them with a metal spatula and bake for another 15 minutes, or until firm and browned. Serve topped with Harissa.

BEANS

Researchers have found that premenopausal women who ate more than about 6 grams of soluble fiber a day (the equivalent of about a single cup of black beans) had 62 percent lower odds of breast cancer compared with women who consumed less than around 4 grams a day. Meanwhile, the American Institute for Cancer Research sifted through some half a million studies and created a landmark scientific consensus report reviewed by twenty-one of the top cancer researchers in the world. One of their summary cancer prevention recommendations is to eat whole grains and/or legumes (beans, split peas, chickpeas, or lentils) with every meal.[127] Not every week or every day. *With every meal!*

Daily Dozen Foods

X BEANS   X OTHER VEGETABLES   X FLAXSEEDS   X NUTS AND SEEDS   X HERBS AND SPICES   X WHOLE GRAINS

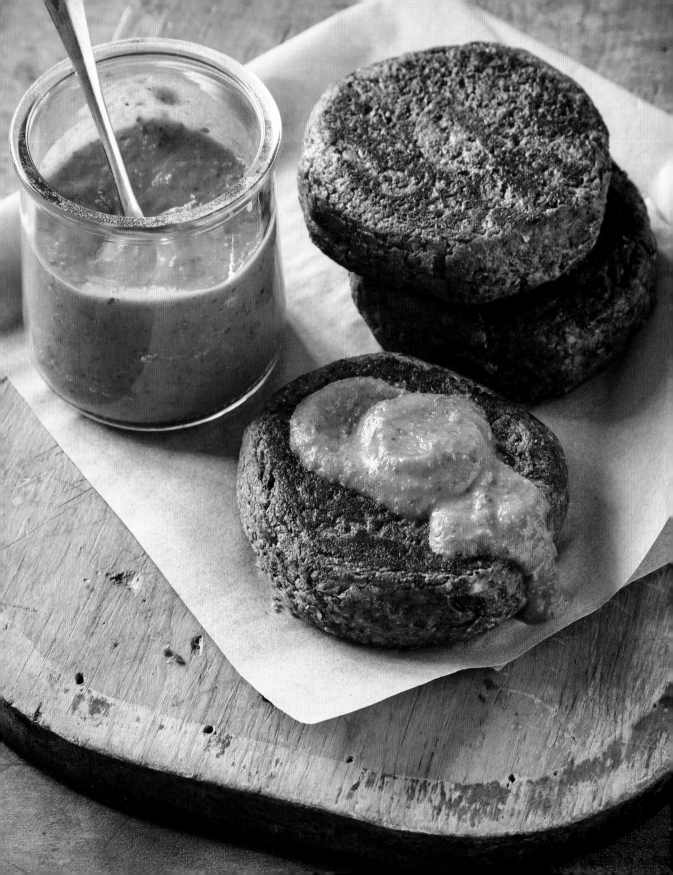

MAC & CHEESE

VEGETABLE UNFRIED RICE

BUCKWHEAT SOBA & EDAMAME WITH ALMOND BUTTER SAUCE

QUINOA PILAF WITH CARROTS & CHICKPEAS

WHOLE WHEAT PASTA WITH LENTIL BOLOGNESE

YELLOW RICE & BLACK BEANS WITH BROCCOLI

STUFFED WINTER SQUASH WITH BLACK BEAN SAUCE

RED QUINOA LOAF WITH GOLDEN GRAVY

HOPPIN' JOHN STUFFED COLLARD ROLLS

ARUGULA PESTO PASTA WITH ROASTED VEGETABLES

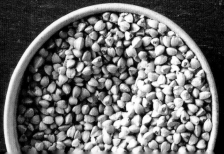

NINE

GREAT GRAINS

Why limit yourself to plain old white rice when there are scores of different whole grains waiting for you to enjoy with tremendous flavor (and many more health benefits)? Some of my favorites are brown, red, or black rice. Yes, they have longer cooking times, which is why I often cook up large batches, portion, and freeze them so I can quickly thaw, prepare, and dig in. As you look through these dishes, keep in mind that other whole grains like barley, buckwheat, millet, freekeh, and oats can be used interchangeably in these recipes. I've also included some fantastic whole-grain pasta options for you.

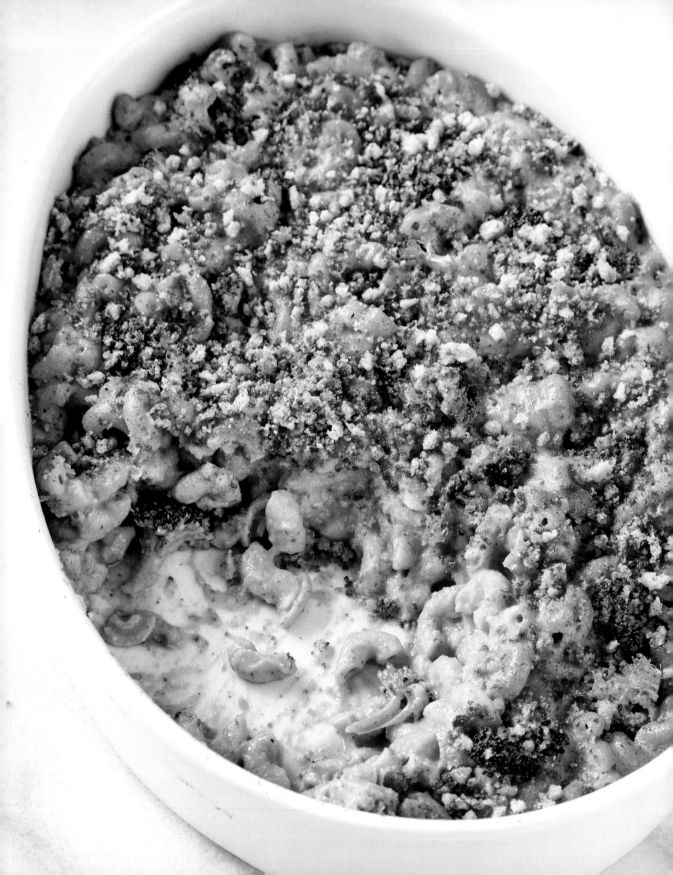

MAC & CHEESE

MAKES: *4* (1½-CUP) SERVINGS · DIFFICULTY: *easy*

Comfort food extraordinaire! If you want to make a stovetop version of this dish, prepare as directed, but instead of baking in the oven, combine everything except the bread crumbs and ¼ teaspoon of the smoked paprika in a pot and heat over medium heat until hot, stirring so it doesn't burn. Sprinkle on the bread crumbs, top with the smoked paprika, and serve.

3 cups Vegetable Broth (page 6)

½ cup chopped red onion

1 garlic clove, chopped

1½ cups chopped carrot or butternut squash

8 ounces 100% whole-grain or bean-based macaroni or other bite-sized pasta

½ cup nutritional yeast

2 tablespoons almond butter

2 teaspoons blended peeled lemon (see page 3)

2 teaspoons white miso paste

1 teaspoon salt-free stone-ground mustard

½ teaspoon smoked paprika

¼ teaspoon fresh turmeric, grated (or ¼ teaspoon ground)

1 teaspoon Savory Spice Blend (page 4), or to taste

1 cup steamed chopped greens or small broccoli florets, liquid pressed out

¼ cup whole-grain bread crumbs

In a large saucepan, heat 1 cup of the broth over medium-high heat. Add the onion, garlic, and carrot. Cover and cook until the vegetables are very soft, 8 to 10 minutes. Remove from the heat and set aside.

Cook the macaroni according to the package instructions until it is al dente. Drain well and set aside.

Preheat the oven to 375°F.

In a high-speed blender, combine the cooked vegetables, the remaining 2 cups of broth, and the nutritional yeast, almond butter, lemon, miso, mustard, ¼ teaspoon of the paprika, the turmeric, and Savory Spice Blend. Blend until very smooth. Taste and adjust the seasonings, if necessary.

Combine the sauce with the drained macaroni, stirring gently to combine. Stir in the cooked greens. Transfer to a 2½-quart baking dish. Sprinkle with the bread crumbs and the remaining ¼ teaspoon of paprika. Bake until hot and golden on top, about 20 minutes. Serve hot.

Daily Dozen Foods

X CRUCIFEROUS VEGETABLES   X OTHER VEGETABLES   X NUTS AND SEEDS   X HERBS AND SPICES   X WHOLE GRAINS

VEGETABLE UNFRIED RICE

MAKES: *4* (2-CUP) SERVINGS · DIFFICULTY: *easy*

Here's a healthy, super-easy take on a classic, and the perfect dish to make with your leftover rice and veggies. What other meal can you prepare with cold cooked rice and whichever vegetables you have on hand? You can also tailor it to suit your taste by upping (or lowering) the spice.

2 tablespoons Umami Sauce (page 5)

1 tablespoon tahini

1 teaspoon white miso paste

1 teaspoon rice vinegar

¼ to ½ teaspoon red pepper flakes (optional)

1 red onion, finely chopped

1 large carrot, shredded

2 cups small broccoli florets

2 garlic cloves, minced

2 to 3 teaspoons grated fresh ginger

3 scallions, minced

3 cups cold cooked brown, red, or black rice

1 cup green peas

In a small bowl, combine the Umami Sauce, tahini, miso, vinegar, and red pepper flakes (if using). Stir in ¼ cup of water and set aside.

Heat ¼ cup of water in a large skillet or wok over medium-high heat. Add the onion and carrot, and cook, stirring, until softened, about 5 minutes. Add the broccoli, garlic, ginger, and scallions and cook for 4 minutes, continuing to stir. Add the rice, peas, and Umami Sauce mixture. Cook, stirring until hot and well combined, about 5 minutes. Serve immediately.

Daily Dozen Foods

✗ CRUCIFEROUS VEGETABLES   ✗ OTHER VEGETABLES   ✗ NUTS AND SEEDS   ✗ HERBS AND SPICES   ✗ WHOLE GRAINS

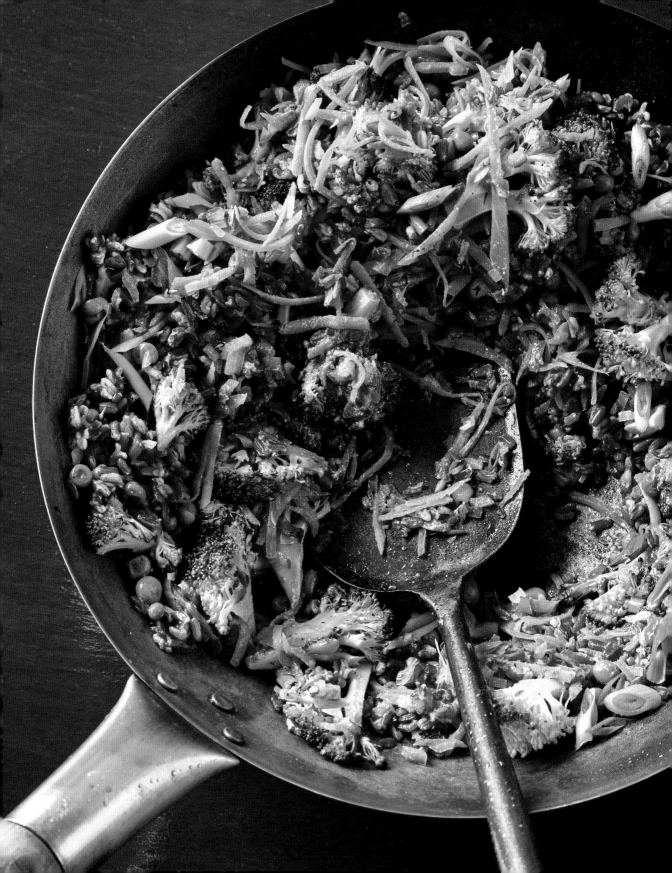

BUCKWHEAT SOBA & EDAMAME WITH ALMOND BUTTER SAUCE

MAKES: *4* (1½-CUP) SERVINGS · DIFFICULTY: *easy*

Buckwheat is another of my mother's favorite foods. Most mornings, she starts her day with kasha, or roasted buckwheat, as a hot cereal, and adds berries and Ceylon cinnamon. There are plenty of other uses for buckwheat as well, especially as soba noodles. (*Soba* is the Japanese term for "buckwheat.")

¼ cup almond butter

1 garlic clove, chopped

2 teaspoons minced fresh ginger

2 tablespoons Umami Sauce (page 5)

½ teaspoon red pepper flakes, or to taste

1 tablespoon blended peeled lime (see page 3)

1 tablespoon white miso paste

8 ounces 100% soba noodles

1 cup frozen shelled edamame, thawed

1 red bell pepper, cut into thin strips

1 carrot, shredded

3 scallions, chopped

1 tablespoon sesame seeds

In a blender or food processor, combine the almond butter, garlic, ginger, Umami Sauce, red pepper flakes, lime, miso, and ⅔ cup of water. Blend until smooth. Set aside.

Cook the soba according to the package directions, adding the edamame to cook with the soba noodles. Drain and run the noodles and edamame under cold water. Transfer to a serving bowl and add the bell pepper, carrot, and scallions. Stir the sauce into the noodles and vegetables, tossing gently to coat. Taste and adjust the seasonings, if needed. Sprinkle with the sesame seeds and serve at room temperature.

VARIATIONS: Replace the edamame with diced cooked tempeh. Use peanut butter or tahini in place of the almond butter.

NUTS

Sometimes it feels like there just aren't enough hours in a day to get everything done. So, instead of trying to make your day longer, why not make your life longer by an extra two years? That's about how long your life span may be increased by eating nuts regularly—one handful (or about a quarter of a cup) five or more days a week.[128] Just that one simple and delicious act alone may extend your life.

Daily Dozen Foods

✗ BEANS ✗ OTHER VEGETABLES ✗ NUTS AND SEEDS ✗ HERBS AND SPICES ✗ WHOLE GRAINS

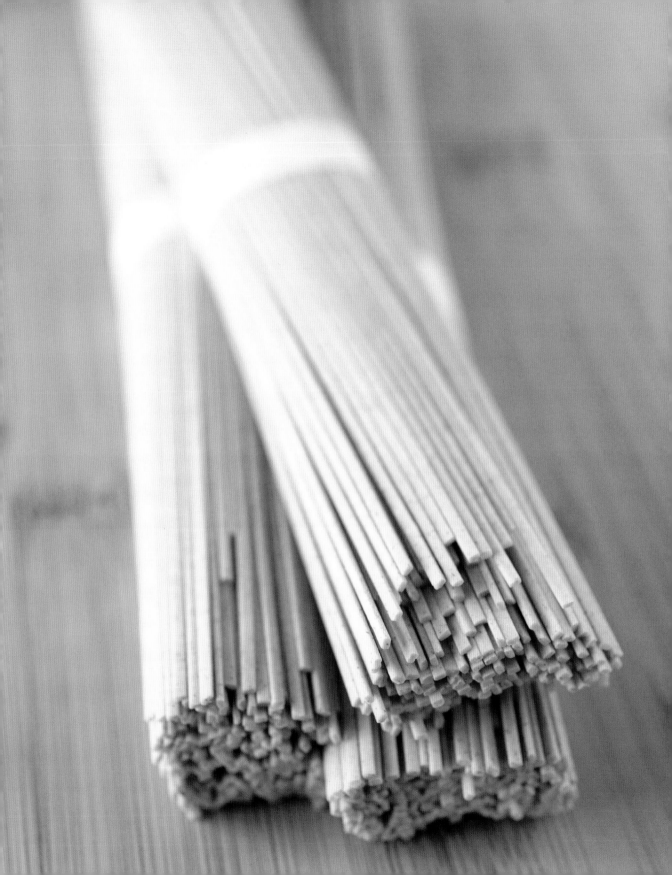

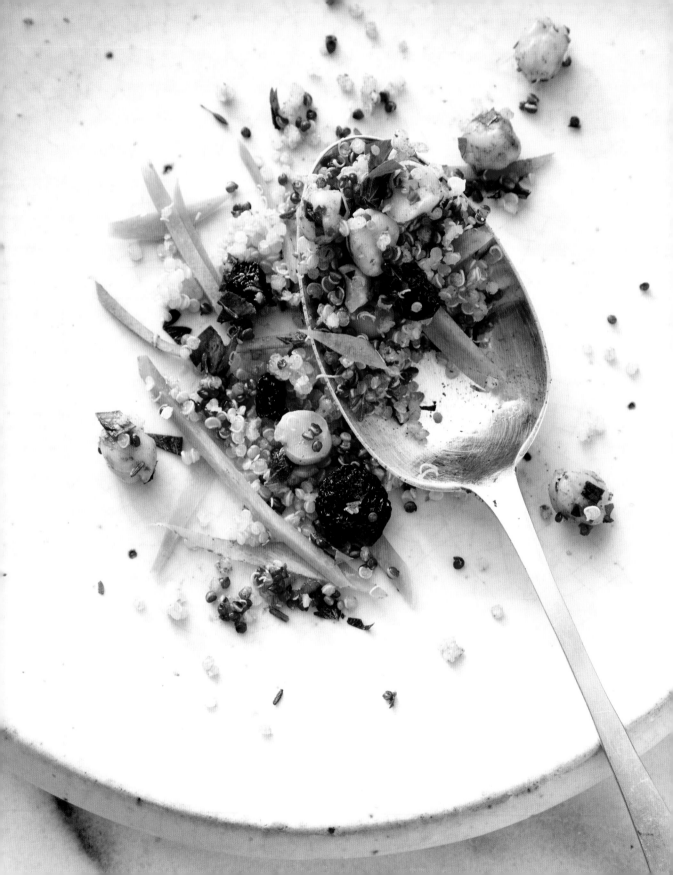

QUINOA PILAF WITH CARROTS & CHICKPEAS

MAKES: *4* (1½-CUP) SERVINGS · DIFFICULTY: *easy*

Brown, red, or black rice, whole wheat couscous, or another whole grain may be used instead of the quinoa—just adjust the cooking time accordingly.

1 cup quinoa, well rinsed and drained

2 teaspoons blended peeled lemon (see page 3)

1 teaspoon date sugar

1 teaspoon cumin seeds

1 teaspoon smoked paprika

1 teaspoon white miso paste

1 teaspoon Savory Spice Blend (page 4), or to taste

3 carrots, shredded

1½ cups cooked or 1 15.5-ounce BPA-free can or Tetra Pak salt-free chickpeas, drained and rinsed

1 cup peas

⅓ cup raisins

¼ cup minced fresh cilantro or parsley

Bring 2 cups of water to a boil in a saucepan. Add the quinoa and lower the heat to a simmer. Cover and cook until the quinoa is tender and the water is absorbed, about 15 minutes. Set aside.

In a large bowl, whisk together the lemon, date sugar, cumin seeds, paprika, miso, and Savory Spice Blend. Add the quinoa, carrots, chickpeas, and peas and toss to coat. Add the raisins and cilantro and toss again to combine. Serve immediately. Alternatively, you can serve this pilaf chilled—just cover and refrigerate for 1 to 2 hours before serving.

Daily Dozen Foods

✗ BEANS   ✗ OTHER VEGETABLES   ✗ HERBS AND SPICES   ✗ WHOLE GRAINS

WHOLE WHEAT PASTA WITH LENTIL BOLOGNESE

MAKES: *4* (2-CUP) SERVINGS · DIFFICULTY: *easy*

This sauce has it all—veggies, herbs, spice, protein, and much more. Don't limit yourself to enjoying it only with pasta. It's delicious on a bed of cooked greens; over brown, black, or red rice; or as a stuffing for bell peppers.

1 28-ounce jar or Tetra Pak salt-free diced tomatoes, undrained

1 medium red onion, finely chopped

3 garlic cloves, minced

8 ounces cremini mushrooms, finely chopped

¼ cup jarred tomato paste

1 tablespoon white miso paste

2 tablespoons nutritional yeast

1½ teaspoons dried basil

1 teaspoon dried oregano

½ teaspoon red pepper flakes

½ teaspoon date sugar

1½ cups cooked or canned lentils

8 ounces 100% whole-grain or bean-based spaghetti

Nutty Parm (page 4)

Pour the liquid from the jar of tomatoes into a large skillet over medium heat. Set the tomatoes aside for now. Add the onion and garlic and cook, stirring occasionally, until softened, about 5 minutes. Add the mushrooms and cook for 2 minutes longer; then stir in the tomato paste, miso, nutritional yeast, basil, oregano, red pepper flakes, and date sugar. Stir in 1 cup of water, and then add the tomatoes and lentils, and simmer, stirring frequently, for 15 minutes, or until the sauce has thickened and the flavors have blended, adding a little more water, if desired. Taste and adjust the seasonings, if needed. Keep warm over low heat.

While the sauce is simmering, cook the spaghetti in a large pot of boiling water, stirring occasionally, until it is al dente. To serve, top the pasta with the sauce and sprinkle with Nutty Parm. Serve hot.

Daily Dozen Foods

✗ BEANS   ✗ OTHER VEGETABLES   ✗ NUTS AND SEEDS   ✗ HERBS AND SPICES   ✗ WHOLE GRAINS

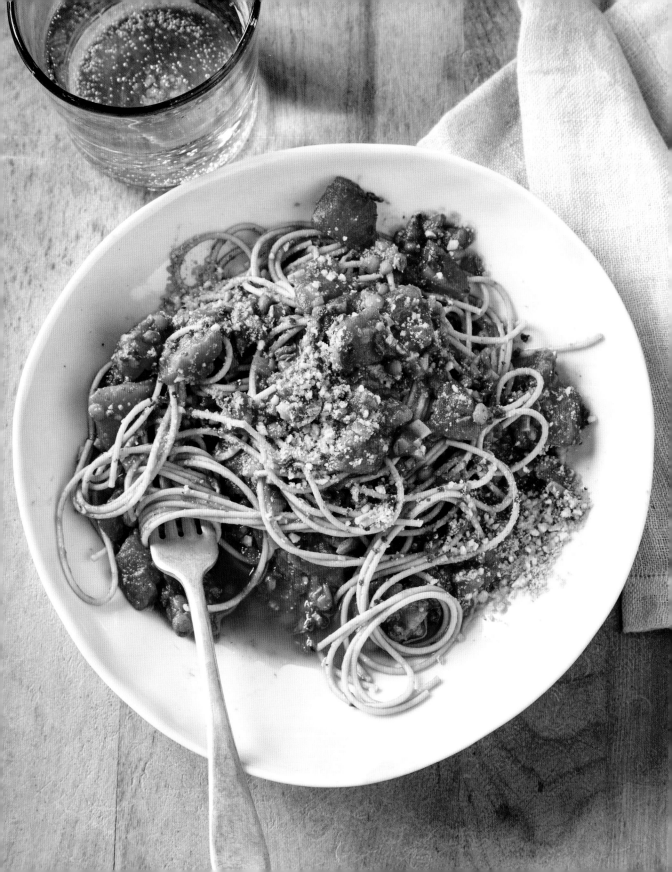

YELLOW RICE & BLACK BEANS WITH BROCCOLI

MAKES: *4* (1¼-CUP) SERVINGS · DIFFICULTY: *easy*

If you prefer, use white beans instead of black beans. I like to add chopped tomatoes and minced scallions just before serving for an extra oomph of color and zest.

1 large shallot, minced

1 teaspoon minced fresh ginger

2 teaspoons white miso paste

2 tablespoons nutritional yeast

1 ¼-inch piece fresh turmeric, grated (or ¼ teaspoon ground)

½ teaspoon ground coriander

¼ teaspoon ground cumin

⅛ teaspoon cayenne pepper

1 cup long-grain brown, red, or black rice

2½ cups Vegetable Broth (page 6) or water

3 cups small broccoli florets

1½ cups cooked or 1 15.5-ounce BPA-free can or Tetra Pak salt-free black beans, drained and rinsed

Heat 2 tablespoons of water in a large skillet or saucepan over medium-high heat. Add the shallots and ginger and cook for 1 minute. Stir in the miso, nutritional yeast, turmeric, coriander, cumin, cayenne, and rice. Stir in the broth and bring to a boil. Lower the heat to a simmer, cover, and cook for 35 to 40 minutes, stirring occasionally, or until the rice is just tender. Stir in the broccoli and a little more broth, if needed. Cook for 10 minutes longer, or until the water is absorbed and the broccoli and rice are tender. Stir in the beans and remove from the heat. Serve hot.

Daily Dozen Foods

X BEANS   *X* CRUCIFEROUS VEGETABLES   *X* HERBS AND SPICES   *X* WHOLE GRAINS

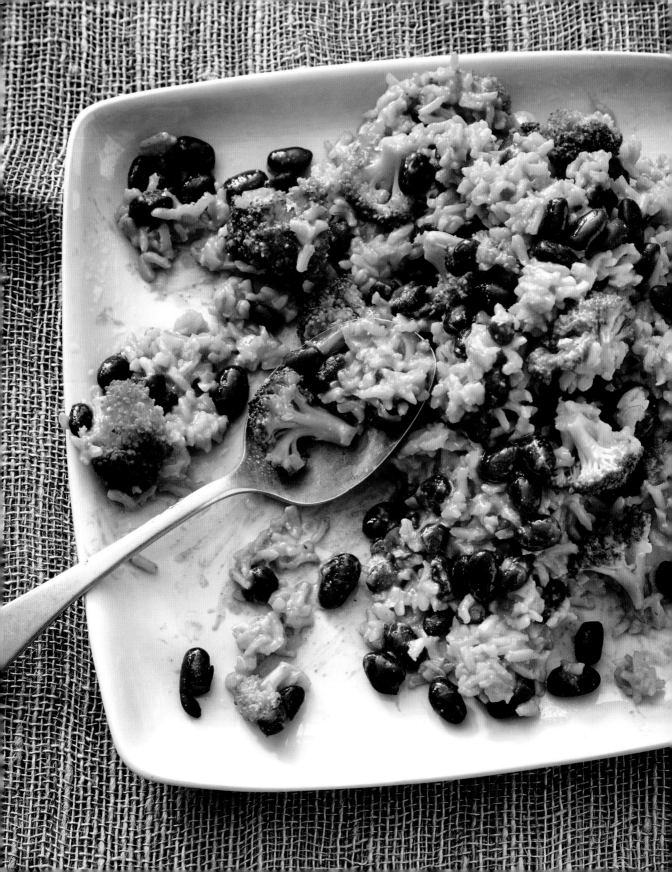

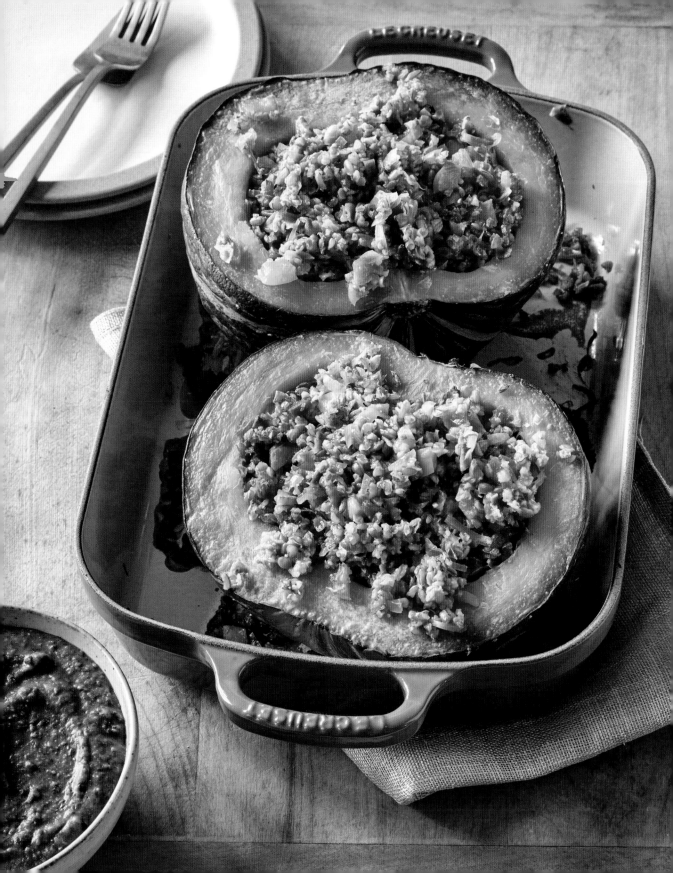

STUFFED WINTER SQUASH WITH BLACK BEAN SAUCE

MAKES: *4* SERVINGS · DIFFICULTY: *moderate*

If you can't find a squash large enough for stuffing, you can cut the squash into ½-inch-thick slices, roast them, and then arrange them in a baking dish, topped with the stuffing. Cover and bake at 350°F for 30 minutes and serve with the sauce drizzled on top.

1 large winter squash (such as buttercup or kabocha), halved and seeded

STUFFING

1 small red onion, chopped

2 cups finely chopped purple cabbage

2 garlic cloves, minced

1 small red, green, orange, or yellow bell pepper, chopped

2¼ cups Vegetable Broth (page 6)

1 tablespoon white miso paste

2 tablespoons nutritional yeast

1 cup bulgur

BLACK BEAN SAUCE

½ cup Vegetable Broth (page 6)

2 garlic cloves, minced

1½ cups cooked or 1 15.5-ounce BPA-free can or Tetra Pak salt-free black beans, drained and rinsed

2 tablespoons Umami Sauce (page 5)

1 tablespoon white miso paste

1 tablespoon jarred tomato paste

2 tablespoons nutritional yeast

½ teaspoon ground cumin

1 teaspoon ground coriander

⅛ to ¼ teaspoon cayenne pepper

Preheat the oven to 375°F. Arrange the squash halves, cut side down, in a shallow baking pan. Add ¼ inch of water to the pan and cover tightly. Bake for 20 minutes to soften slightly.

STUFFING: Heat ¼ cup of water in a large skillet over medium heat. Add the onion, cabbage, garlic, and bell pepper. Cover and cook until softened, about 4 minutes. Stir in the broth, miso, nutritional yeast, and bulgur. Bring to a boil, then reduce the heat to low, and simmer 5 minutes longer. Remove from the heat and let it sit, covered, for 10 minutes, or until the water is absorbed by the bulgur.

Turn over the squash halves so they are cut side up and fill them with the stuffing, packing them well. Cover and bake until the squash is tender, about 30 minutes.

SAUCE: While the stuffed squash is baking, make the sauce. In a saucepan, combine the broth and garlic, and bring to a boil. Lower the heat to a simmer and stir in the beans, Umami Sauce, miso, tomato paste, nutritional yeast, cumin, coriander, and cayenne. Simmer for 5 minutes; then transfer to a blender or food processor and blend until smooth, adding a little more broth, if needed, for the desired consistency. Return the sauce to the saucepan and keep warm over low heat. Taste and adjust the seasonings, if needed. To serve, top the baked squash with the sauce and serve hot.

Daily Dozen Foods

X BEANS   X CRUCIFEROUS VEGETABLES   X OTHER VEGETABLES   X HERBS AND SPICES   X WHOLE GRAINS

RED QUINOA LOAF WITH GOLDEN GRAVY

MAKES: *6* SERVINGS · DIFFICULTY: *moderate*

I like to serve this dish on a bed of cooked greens. If you can't find red quinoa, look for black quinoa or, in a pinch, regular. It's also fantastic over black, red, or brown rice.

QUINOA LOAF

1 small red onion, coarsely chopped

1 garlic clove, crushed

½ cup walnuts

1 cup mushrooms, quartered

1½ cups cooked or 1 15.5-ounce BPA-free can or Tetra Pak salt-free dark red kidney beans, drained and rinsed

1 cup cooked red quinoa

½ cup old-fashioned rolled oats

2 tablespoons tahini or peanut butter

2 tablespoons nutritional yeast

2 tablespoons ground flaxseeds

1 tablespoon minced fresh parsley

1 tablespoon white miso paste

1 teaspoon smoked paprika

½ teaspoon dried thyme

½ teaspoon dried sage

½ teaspoon dried basil

¼ teaspoon ground black pepper

QUINOA LOAF: Preheat the oven to 350°F. Line a loaf pan with a piece of parchment paper the same length of the loaf pan and long enough to come up and over the sides by an inch or two. (For an 8 × 4 × 2½-inch loaf pan, your parchment paper should be about 8 × 11 inches.)

Combine the onion, garlic, and walnuts in a food processor and pulse until finely minced. Add the mushrooms and beans and pulse until finely chopped and well combined. Add the remaining loaf ingredients and process until well combined. If the mixture seems too wet to hold together, add more oats. If the mixture seems too dry, add a little water.

Transfer the mixture into the prepared loaf pan. Press firmly into the pan, smoothing the top. Bake until firm and golden brown, 50 to 60 minutes. Check at around 40 minutes: if the top of the loaf is getting too brown, cover with foil for the last 10 to 20 minutes of baking time.

Daily Dozen Foods

✗ BEANS   ✗ FLAXSEEDS   ✗ NUTS AND SEEDS   ✗ HERBS AND SPICES   ✗ WHOLE GRAINS

GOLDEN GRAVY

⅓ cup Vegetable Broth (page 6)

2 garlic cloves, minced

1½ cups cooked or 1 15.5-ounce BPA-free can or Tetra Pak salt-free chickpeas, drained and rinsed

2 tablespoons nutritional yeast

1 tablespoon white miso paste

1 teaspoon dried thyme

1 ¼-inch piece fresh turmeric, grated (or ¼ teaspoon ground)

¼ teaspoon ground black pepper

GOLDEN GRAVY: While the loaf is baking, make the gravy. In a saucepan, combine the broth and garlic and bring to a boil. Lower the heat to a simmer and stir in all the remaining gravy ingredients. Simmer for 5 minutes, and then transfer to a blender or food processor and blend until smooth. Return the gravy to the saucepan. Taste and adjust the seasonings, if needed. Keep warm over low heat.

When the loaf is done baking, remove it from the oven, uncover, and let sit for 10 minutes before slicing. Top with the gravy. Serve hot.

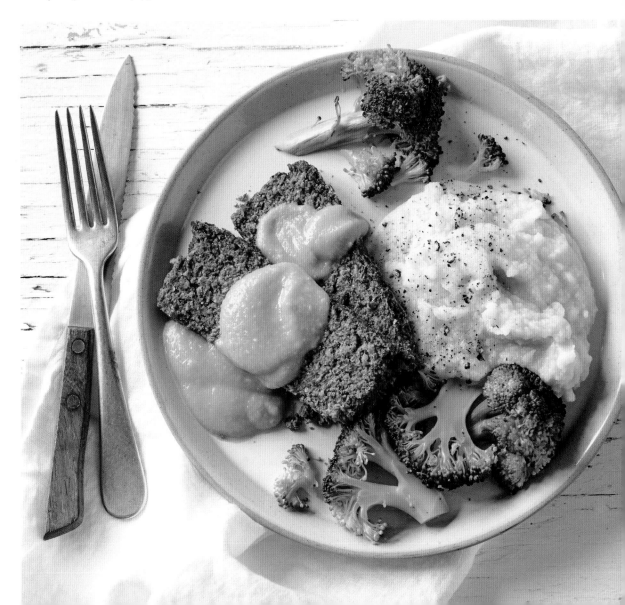

HOPPIN' JOHN STUFFED COLLARD ROLLS

MAKES: *4* TO *6* SERVINGS (2 ROLLS PER SERVING) · DIFFICULTY: *moderate*

This Southern riff on stuffed cabbage rolls take some time to assemble, but it is more than worth the effort. For an easier variation, cook the collard greens until tender, then chop and stir them into the rice mixture, add the remaining ingredients, and heat until hot.

1 14.5-ounce BPA-free can or Tetra Pak salt-free diced tomatoes, undrained

1 red onion, minced

1 green bell pepper, minced

3 garlic cloves, minced

1 teaspoon smoked paprika

½ teaspoon dried thyme

¼ teaspoon cayenne pepper

¼ teaspoon ground black pepper

1½ cups cooked brown, black, or red rice

1½ cups cooked or 1 15.5-ounce BPA-free can or Tetra Pak salt-free black-eyed peas, drained and rinsed

8 to 12 collard leaves, well washed, ends trimmed

1 teaspoon Healthy Hot Sauce (page 8), or to taste

2 tablespoons nutritional yeast

1 teaspoon white miso paste

Pour the tomato liquid into a large, nonstick skillet over medium-high heat, setting the tomatoes aside. Add the onion, cover, and cook for 3 minutes to soften. Stir in the bell pepper and garlic and cook 3 minutes longer or until soft, adding a little water, if needed, so they don't burn. Stir in the paprika, thyme, cayenne, and black pepper. Add the cooked rice and black-eyed peas. Reduce the heat to low and cook for about 10 minutes, stirring frequently, to mix well and blend the flavors. Remove from the heat and set aside.

Bring a large pot of water to boil. Place one of the collard leaves, stem side up, on a flat work surface. Use a sharp knife to remove as much of the thick central rib as you can without cutting through the leaf. Repeat with the remaining leaves. Working in batches, place the collard leaves into the boiling water, pressing them down to keep them submerged. Boil for about 3 minutes. Remove the leaves from the pot with a slotted spoon and rinse under cool water. Preheat the oven to 350°F.

In a bowl, combine the reserved diced tomatoes with the Healthy Hot Sauce, nutritional yeast, and miso, stirring to blend. Spoon half of the seasoned tomatoes onto the bottom of a large, shallow baking dish and set aside. On a flat work surface, place a collard leaf with its stem end nearest you. Place about 3 tablespoons of the rice mixture about a quarter of the way from the bottom of the collard leaf. Fold the sides of the leaf over the middle and then fold the stem end over the filling, tucking it in behind the filling. Roll up tightly and carefully place it into the baking dish. Repeat until all of the rolls are prepared. Spoon the remaining seasoned tomato mixture over the rolls. Tightly cover the baking dish and bake for 50 to 60 minutes, or until the rolls are tender. Serve hot.

Daily Dozen Foods

✗ **GREENS**   ✗ **OTHER VEGETABLES**   ✗ **HERBS AND SPICES**   ✗ **WHOLE GRAINS**

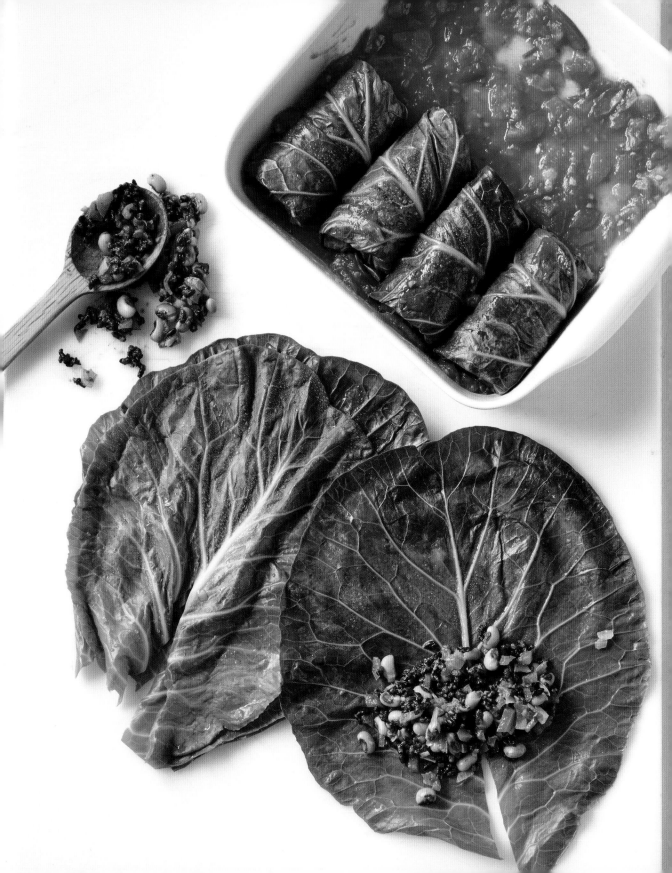

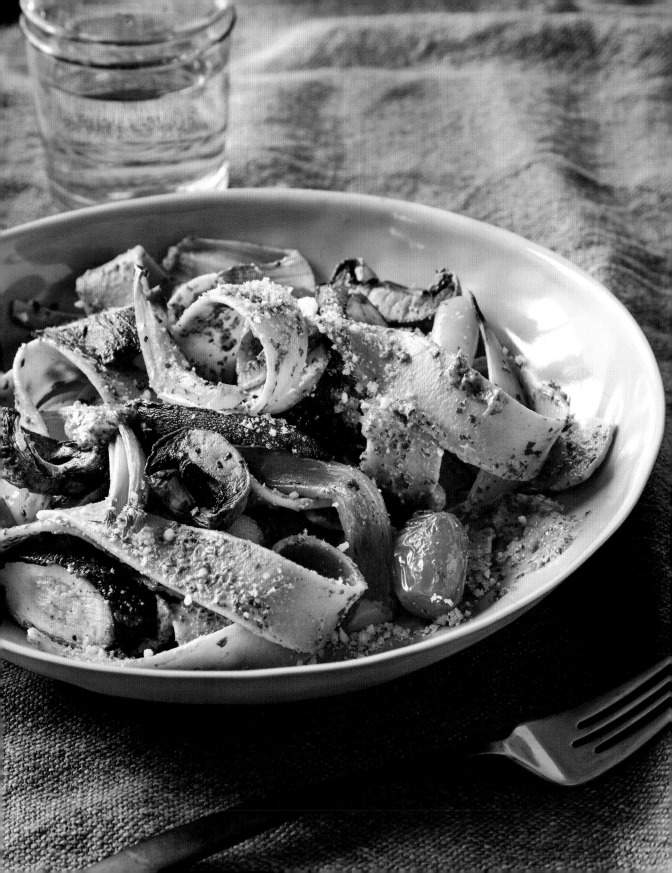

ARUGULA PESTO PASTA WITH ROASTED VEGETABLES

MAKES: *4* (2-CUP) SERVINGS · DIFFICULTY: *easy*

For a variation, omit the pasta and serve on a bed of red, black, or brown rice or another one of your favorite whole grains.

3 garlic cloves

3 cups fresh arugula or spinach

1 cup fresh basil leaves

2 tablespoons tahini

2 tablespoons white miso

1 tablespoon brown rice vinegar

4 shallots, halved or quartered

1 large red or yellow bell pepper, cut into large dice

2 zucchini, trimmed and cut into ½-inch slices

8 white mushrooms

8 cherry tomatoes

¼ teaspoon onion powder

¼ teaspoon garlic powder

¼ teaspoon ground black pepper

8 ounces whole-grain pasta, bean noodles, or your favorite spiralized vegetable noodles

Nutty Parm (page 4)

Chop the garlic in a food processor. Add the arugula and basil, and process until minced. Add the tahini, miso, and vinegar, and continue to process until smooth and creamy. Transfer to a small bowl and set aside.

Preheat the oven to 425°F. Line a large baking sheet with a silicone mat or parchment paper and set aside. Place the shallots, bell pepper, zucchini, mushrooms, and tomatoes in a large bowl and sprinkle with the onion powder, garlic powder, and black pepper, tossing to coat. Transfer the seasoned vegetables to the prepared baking sheet and place in a single layer. Roast the vegetables until tender, 20 to 25 minutes, turning once about halfway through.

While the vegetables are roasting, cook the pasta in a pot of boiling water according to the package directions. Drain the pasta, reserving ½ cup of the cooking liquid. Transfer the pasta to a large, shallow bowl. Blend the hot pasta liquid with the arugula pesto and add to the pasta, tossing to coat. Top with the roasted vegetables and sprinkle with Nutty Parm to taste. Serve hot.

Daily Dozen Foods

✗ GREENS   ✗ OTHER VEGETABLES   ✗ NUTS AND SEEDS   ✗ HERBS AND SPICES   ✗ WHOLE GRAINS

TEN

SIDES

If you're looking for more ways to prepare vegetables, this is the place. For greens that are loaded with flavor, try the Garlic Greens Sauté, the Indian-Style Spinach & Tomatoes, or the Roasted Beets with Balsamic-Braised Beet Greens. The Cauliflower Mash is used to top the Lentil Shepherd's Pie on page 133, but it's also a great side dish in its own right. No one will ever say vegetables are boring when they try the Stuffed Sweet Potatoes with Balsamic-Date Glaze, Buffalo Cauliflower with Ranch Dressing, or the Baked Onion Rings.

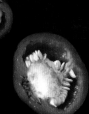

ROASTED ASPARAGUS WITH
YELLOW PEPPER BÉARNAISE

LEMON-ROASTED BRUSSELS SPROUTS
& CARROTS WITH PECANS

ROASTED BEETS WITH
BALSAMIC-BRAISED BEET GREENS

INDIAN-STYLE SPINACH & TOMATOES

PURPLE CABBAGE SAUTÉ

CAULIFLOWER MASH

STUFFED SWEET POTATOES
WITH BALSAMIC-DATE GLAZE

GARLIC GREENS SAUTÉ

BAKED ONION RINGS

BUFFALO CAULIFLOWER
WITH RANCH DRESSING

ROASTED ASPARAGUS WITH YELLOW PEPPER BÉARNAISE

MAKES: *4* (⅔- TO 1-CUP) SERVINGS · DIFFICULTY: *easy*

Once you've roasted asparagus, you may never want to make it any other way. This healthy interpretation of béarnaise sauce—which is typically made with heavy cream, artery-clogging clarified butter, and egg yolk—is also delicious over steamed broccoli, roasted cauliflower, and baked sweet potatoes.

2 cups Vegetable Broth (page 6)

2 shallots, chopped

1 garlic clove, crushed

2 yellow bell peppers, seeded and chopped

1 teaspoon dried tarragon

2 teaspoons white miso paste

1 ¼-inch piece fresh turmeric, grated (or ¼ teaspoon ground)

3 tablespoons nutritional yeast

1 tablespoon tarragon vinegar

2 teaspoons blended peeled lemon (see page 3)

16 to 20 ounces asparagus, ends trimmed

Heat the broth in a saucepan over medium heat. Add the shallots and garlic and cook for 2 minutes to soften. Add the bell peppers and bring to a boil. Lower the heat to a simmer. Add the tarragon, miso, and turmeric and cook for 30 minutes, or until the liquid reduces by half. Transfer to a blender. Add the nutritional yeast, vinegar, and lemon, and process until smooth. Return the sauce to the pan and keep warm.

Preheat the oven to 425°F. Line a large baking pan with a silicone mat or parchment paper and place the asparagus in a single layer. Roast the asparagus until it is tender, 10 to 18 minutes, depending on the thickness of the asparagus and how tender you like it. Transfer to a platter and drizzle with the sauce.

Daily Dozen Foods

X OTHER VEGETABLES   X HERBS AND SPICES

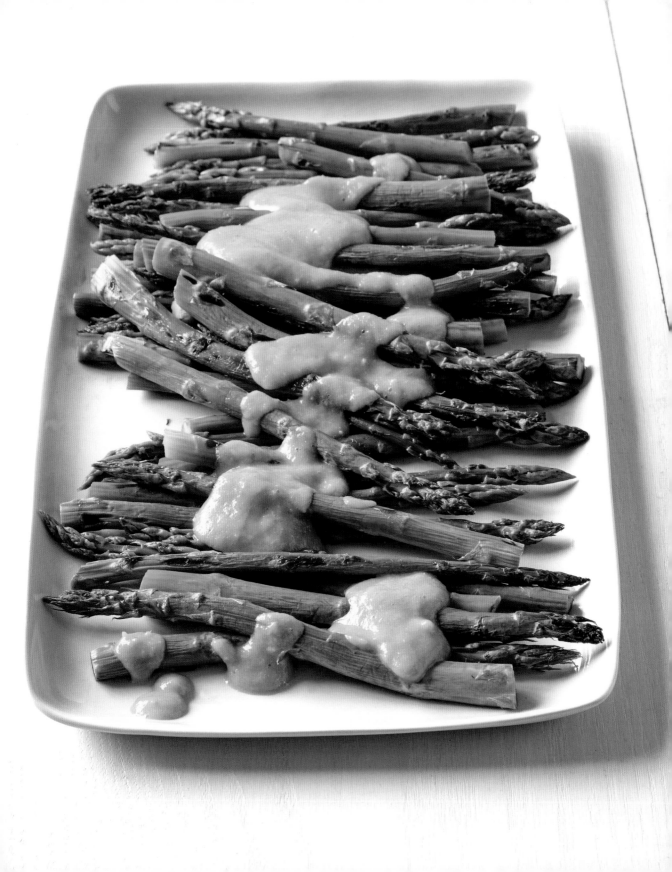

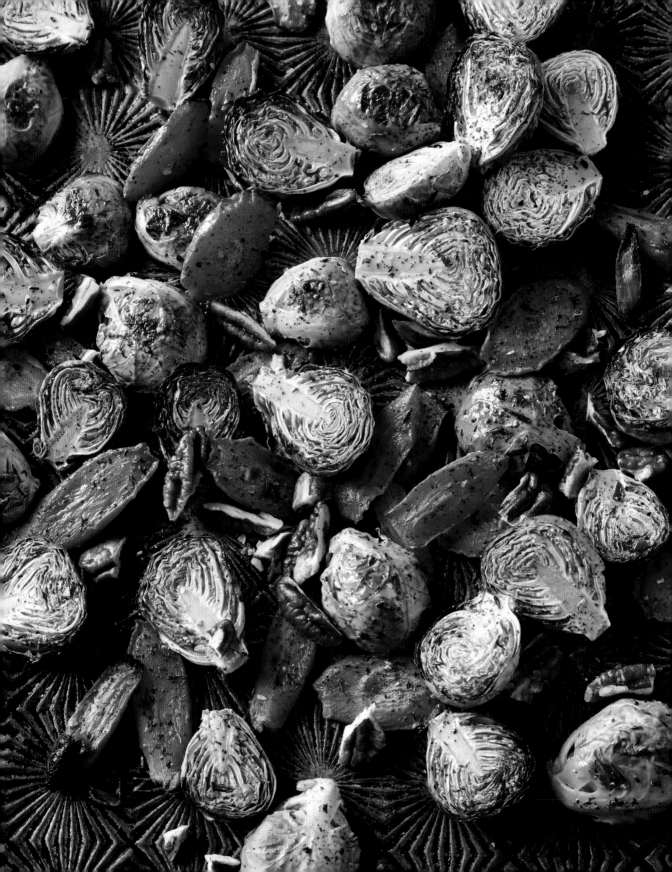

LEMON-ROASTED BRUSSELS SPROUTS & CARROTS WITH PECANS

MAKES: *4* SERVINGS · DIFFICULTY: *easy*

Roasting dramatically improves the flavor of Brussels sprouts. They're even better with the addition of carrots for color, pecans for crunch, and a spritz of lemon to brighten the taste.

1 pound Brussels sprouts, trimmed and halved lengthwise

2 carrots, cut diagonally into ¼-inch slices

2 teaspoons Savory Spice Blend (page 4)

⅓ cup raw pecan pieces

1 tablespoon blended peeled lemon (see page 3)

Preheat the oven to 425°F. Line a large baking pan with a silicone mat or parchment paper and place the Brussels sprouts and carrots in a single layer. Season the vegetables with half of the Savory Spice Blend and roast for 10 minutes. Remove from the oven, stir the vegetables, and then roast for another 5 minutes, or until the vegetables are tender. Remove from the oven once again. Transfer to a platter and sprinkle with the pecans, lemon, and remaining spice blend.

BRUSSELS SPROUTS

Consuming Brussels sprouts (along with cabbage, cauliflower, and broccoli) has been associated with a lower risk of colon cancer in the middle and right side of your body.[129] In vitro, Brussels sprout extracts were found to effectively suppress breast cancer cell growth.[130] Quite a lot of goodness in such a tiny little crucifer!

Daily Dozen Foods

X CRUCIFEROUS VEGETABLES · X OTHER VEGETABLES · X NUTS AND SEEDS · X HERBS AND SPICES

ROASTED BEETS WITH BALSAMIC-BRAISED BEET GREENS

MAKES: *4* (1-CUP) SERVINGS · DIFFICULTY: *easy*

Beets are a concentrated source of vegetable nitrates, which can lower blood pressure and improve blood flow. If you've never been a fan of beets, it may be because you've never had them roasted. The cooking of beet greens with beet root seems almost like a violation of the biblical prohibition against boiling a kid in its mother's milk, but I think we're cool.

1 bunch medium beets with greens

1 red onion, cut into ½-inch wedges

1 teaspoon dried oregano

½ cup balsamic vinegar

2 teaspoons date sugar

1 teaspoon grated orange zest

Ground black pepper

Preheat the oven to 400°F. Remove the greens from the beets, rinse them well, remove and discard any large stems, and set aside. Trim the ends of the beets, leaving the skins on, and scrub the beets well. If any of the beets are large, cut them in half lengthwise. (The beets should be about the same size so as to cook evenly.)

Line a large baking dish with a silicone mat or parchment paper and place the beets and onions in a single layer. Season with the oregano and cover tightly. Roast the vegetables for 30 minutes, then uncover, stir, and return the vegetables to the oven, uncovered, to roast for 10 minutes longer, or until the beets are tender when pierced with a fork.

Finely chop the beet greens and transfer to a skillet with ¼ cup of water. Cook over medium heat, stirring, until the greens are just tender, about 3 minutes. Stir in the balsamic vinegar and date sugar. Increase the heat to medium-high and cook until the vinegar has reduced to a syrup consistency. Remove from the heat.

Remove the vegetables from the oven. Cut the beets into wedges and pull away and discard the outer skin. Transfer the beets and onion to a serving dish, top with the balsamic greens, and add the orange zest, tossing lightly to coat. Sprinkle with black pepper to taste and serve.

Daily Dozen Foods

✗ GREENS   ✗ OTHER VEGETABLES   ✗ HERBS AND SPICES

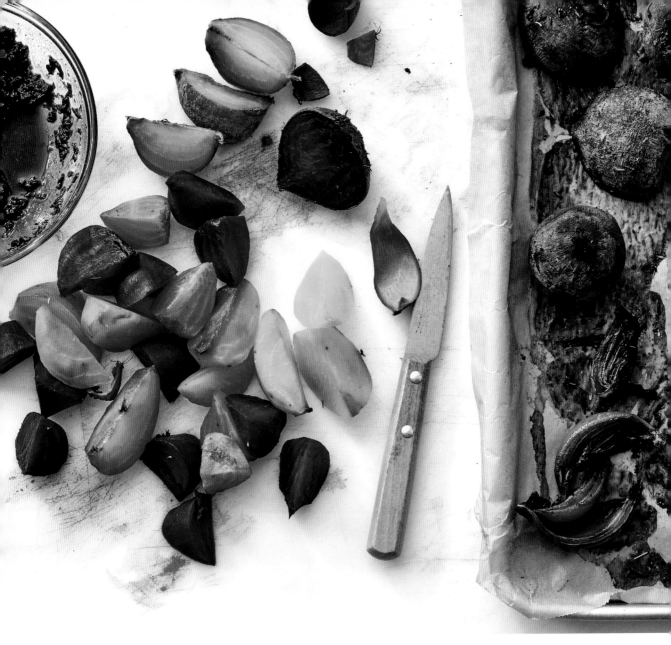

BEETS

In one study, men and women eating 1½ cups of baked beets seventy-five minutes before running a race improved their running performance while maintaining the same heart rate and even reported less exertion.[131] Not trying to improve your splits? Keep loading up on beets, because a 2015 study found that people who consumed a cup of beet juice daily for four weeks reduced their systolic blood pressure by about 8 points.[132]

INDIAN-STYLE SPINACH & TOMATOES

MAKES: *4* (1-CUP) SERVINGS · DIFFICULTY: *easy*

This simple recipe is bursting with flavor. It's great served over quinoa, black, red, or brown rice, or even more greens.

1 pound fresh spinach

1 14.5-ounce BPA-free can or Tetra Pak salt-free diced tomatoes, undrained

8 to 12 ounces cremini mushrooms, sliced

1½ teaspoons grated fresh ginger

1 teaspoon ground coriander

1 ¼-inch piece fresh turmeric, grated (or ¼ teaspoon ground)

¼ teaspoon ground cumin

¼ teaspoon red pepper flakes

1 tablespoon white miso paste

Steam the spinach until tender, 3 to 5 minutes. Drain well, pressing out any excess liquid. Set aside the tomatoes for now. Purée the spinach in a blender or food processor and set aside. Drain the tomato liquid into a large skillet over medium heat. Add the mushrooms, ginger, coriander, turmeric, cumin, and red pepper flakes and cook, stirring, for 1 minute. Stir in the tomatoes and miso and cook for 3 minutes before stirring in the puréed spinach. Continue cooking until the mixture is hot and well blended.

Daily Dozen Foods

✗ GREENS   ✗ OTHER VEGETABLES   ✗ HERBS AND SPICES

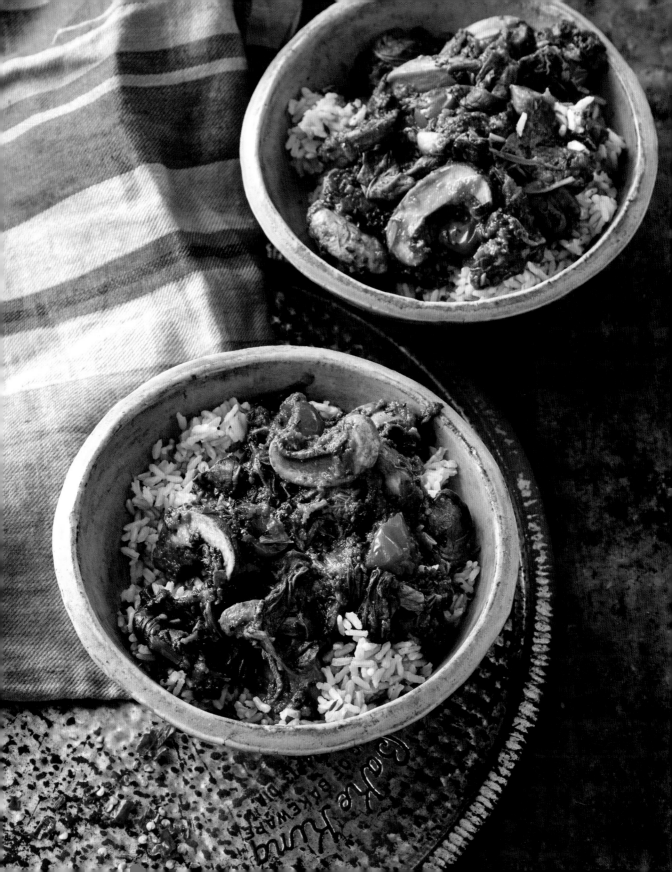

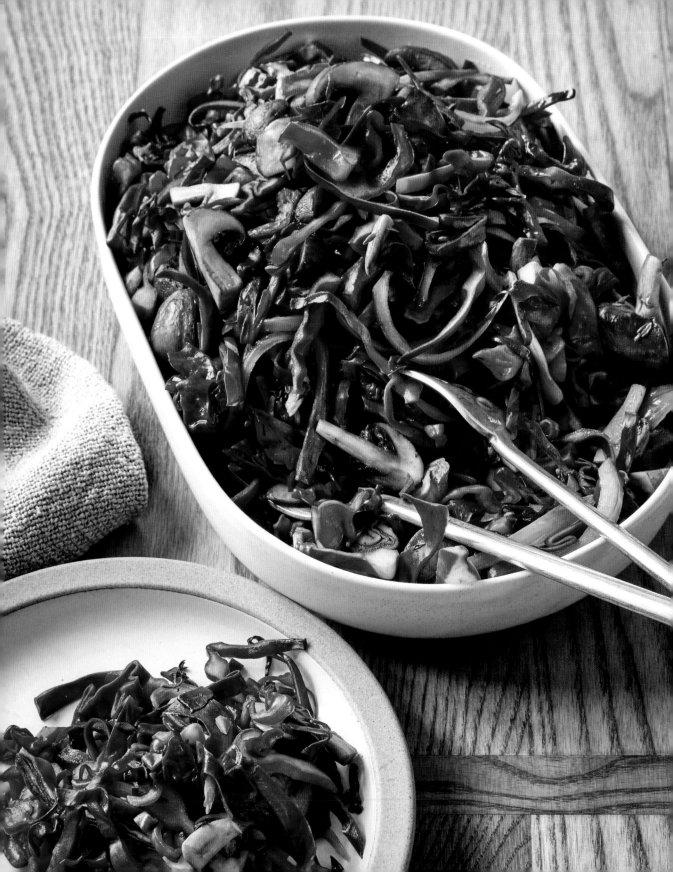

PURPLE CABBAGE SAUTÉ

MAKES: *4* (1⅓-CUP) SERVINGS • DIFFICULTY: *easy*

This cabbage dish is especially good served over braised tempeh.

¼ cup Vegetable Broth (page 6) or water

1 medium red onion, minced

6 cups finely shredded purple cabbage

2 cups chopped mushrooms (any variety)

2 teaspoons minced fresh thyme, or 1 teaspoon dried

3 tablespoons Umami Sauce (page 5)

Ground black pepper

Heat the broth in a medium skillet over medium heat. Add the onion and cabbage and cook, stirring frequently, until the vegetables have softened, about 4 minutes. Add the mushrooms and thyme. Continue to cook, stirring, for about 4 more minutes. Season with the Umami Sauce, tossing to coat. Serve hot sprinkled with black pepper to taste.

Daily Dozen Foods

✗ CRUCIFEROUS VEGETABLES   ✗ OTHER VEGETABLES   ✗ HERBS AND SPICES

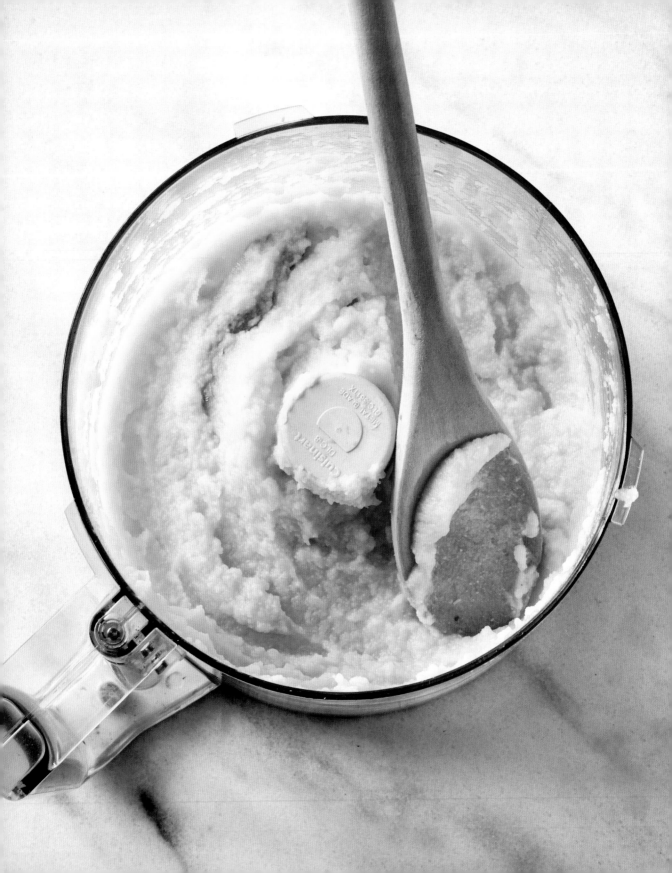

CAULIFLOWER MASH

MAKES: *4* (1-CUP) SERVINGS · DIFFICULTY: *easy*

Enjoy this delightful dish in place of mashed white potatoes or as a topping for the Lentil Shepherd's Pie on page 133.

1 head cauliflower, trimmed and cut into 1-inch pieces

1 tablespoon nutritional yeast

1 teaspoon white miso paste

2 teaspoons Roasted Garlic (page 6) (optional)

Steam the cauliflower until soft, about 10 minutes. Transfer to a bowl or a food processor. Add the nutritional yeast, miso, and Roasted Garlic (if using) and mash or purée until smooth. Serve hot.

Daily Dozen Foods

X CRUCIFEROUS VEGETABLES   X OTHER VEGETABLES

STUFFED SWEET POTATOES WITH BALSAMIC-DATE GLAZE

MAKES: *4* SERVINGS · DIFFICULTY: *easy*

I love sweet potatoes, one of the healthiest foods on the planet. The purple ones are the best, and you can usually find them at Asian markets and specialty natural groceries. They're so good I send them out in the mail as holiday gifts. After all, what is more comforting on a wintry day than a nice, warm, steamy sweet potato? Here's a recipe for a stocking stuffer you can stuff.

4 medium sweet potatoes

½ cup green peas, steamed

2 tablespoons minced fresh chives or scallions

¼ cup raw slivered almonds

Balsamic-Date Glaze (page 8)

Ground black pepper

Preheat the oven to 400°F. Place the sweet potatoes on a baking sheet lined with a silicone mat or parchment paper. Prick each potato with a fork in two or three places and bake until tender, about 1 hour.

When the potatoes are done baking, transfer them to a work surface and allow to cool slightly. Cut each sweet potato in half lengthwise and scoop out the insides of the potatoes into a bowl, leaving about ¼ inch of potato attached to the skin. Add the peas and chives and mix well. Spoon the mixture into each half and return the stuffed sweet potatoes to the oven for about 15 minutes to heat through. Sprinkle with almonds, drizzle with Balsamic-Date Glaze, add a few grinds of black pepper to taste, and serve hot.

PEAS

Like edamame, raw English peas (also known as shell or garden peas) can be a great au naturel snack. I fell in love with peas in the pod when I first picked them off the vine at a farm my brother and I spent time on one summer as kids. They were like candy. Every year, I look forward to the few weeks I can find them fresh. The rest of the year, sugar snap peas can substitute as a good vegetable finger food.

Daily Dozen Foods

✗ OTHER VEGETABLES   ✗ NUTS AND SEEDS

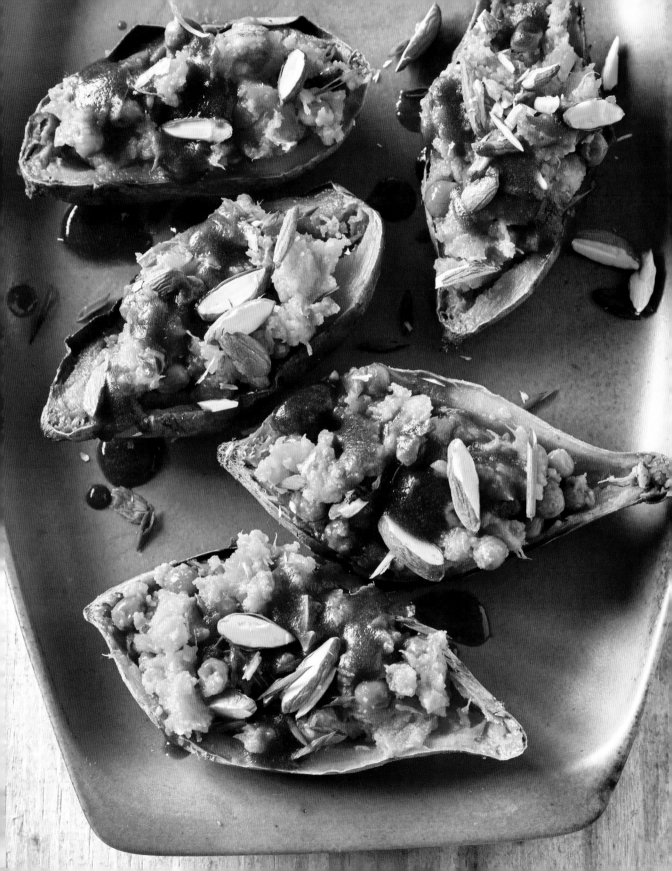

GARLIC GREENS SAUTÉ

MAKES: *4* (¼-CUP) SERVINGS · DIFFICULTY: *easy*

If you wish, transform this recipe into a main dish by adding about 2 cups of cooked white beans and serving over quinoa or black, red, or brown rice, or tossing with 100% whole-grain or bean pasta.

⅓ cup Vegetable Broth (page 6) or water

3 to 4 garlic cloves, minced

1 teaspoon dried basil

½ teaspoon dried oregano

¼ to ½ teaspoon red pepper flakes

2 teaspoons white miso paste

10 to 12 ounces dark leafy greens, tough stems removed, then chopped

Ground black pepper

Combine the broth, garlic, basil, oregano, and red pepper flakes in a large pot and bring to a boil over medium-high heat. Lower the heat to medium and cook for 1 minute to soften the garlic. Stir in the miso and then add the greens, cooking until they wilt, 2 to 6 minutes depending on the type of greens. Serve hot sprinkled with black pepper to taste.

TEN WAYS TO ENJOY GREENS

1. Add raw greens (kale, spinach) to a smoothie.
2. Sauté them (chard, kale, arugula, escarole, spinach) with garlic, raisins, or nuts.
3. Add them (chard, spinach, Asian greens, arugula) to a soup.
4. Steam and top them (kale, spinach) with a sauce.
5. Bake them (kale) into chips.
6. Pair them (chard, collards, spinach, watercress) with beans and whole grains or pasta.
7. Purée them (spinach, watercress, arugula) into a dip or sauce.
8. Add them (spinach, watercress) to a sandwich or salad.
9. Braise them (collards, kale) and drizzle with balsamic vinegar.
10. Stir-fry them (Asian greens, arugula, kale) with ginger and sesame seeds.

Daily Dozen Foods

X GREENS   X HERBS AND SPICES

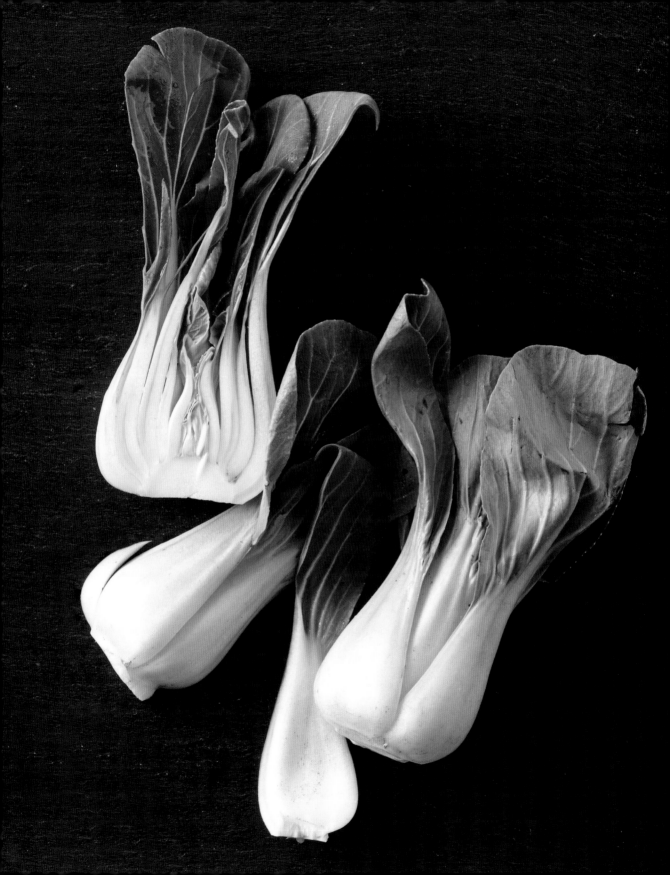

BAKED ONION RINGS

MAKES: *4* SERVINGS (5 ONION RINGS PER SERVING) · DIFFICULTY: *moderate*

Onion rings were a favorite of mine growing up, but I thankfully (and heartfully) gave up my taste for those greasy, oily, deep-fried, fatty monstrosities. The onion rings in this recipe come out pretty close to perfection. Try them with Black Bean Burgers (page 88) and Beet Burgers (98).

1 large red onion, cut into ½-inch-thick slices

⅔ cup oat flour

¼ cup chickpea flour

1 cup Almond Milk (page 2)

1 teaspoon rice vinegar

⅓ cup cornmeal

¾ cup 100% whole-grain salt-free bread crumbs

⅓ cup nutritional yeast

2 tablespoons Savory Spice Blend (page 4)

1 teaspoon smoked paprika

Preheat the oven to 425°F. Line a large baking sheet with a silicone mat or parchment paper and set aside. Separate the onion slices into rings. Transfer to a bowl and set aside.

In a shallow bowl, combine the oat flour, chickpea flour, Almond Milk, and vinegar, stirring to blend well.

In a separate shallow bowl, combine the cornmeal, bread crumbs, nutritional yeast, Savory Spice Blend, and paprika, mixing well.

In a row, line up the bowls of onion rings, batter, and breading mixture, and the prepared baking sheet. Dip an onion ring into the batter, coating it all over. Transfer the onion ring to the breading, tossing to coat. Use a clean, dry hand to sprinkle the breading onto the onion as needed. Place the coated onion ring on the prepared baking sheet and repeat with the remaining ingredients, arranging the rings in a single layer. Use a second baking sheet, if needed. You should have enough batter and breading for about twenty onion rings. Bake for 10 minutes; then remove from the oven and carefully turn over the rings. Bake for about 10 minutes longer, or until crisp and nicely browned. Serve hot.

ONIONS

Colorectal cancer starts out as a polyp, which grows from the inner surface of the colon. A 2006 study found that six months of consuming a phytonutrient called quercetin, which is found in vegetables such as red onions, along with curcumin, an active ingredient of the spice turmeric, were found to decrease the number and size of polyps by more than half among patients with a hereditary form of colorectal cancer.[133] Eating onion along with garlic has also been associated with a significantly lower risk of prostate enlargement (known as BPH).[134]

Daily Dozen Foods

X BEANS   X OTHER VEGETABLES   X HERBS AND SPICES   X WHOLE GRAINS

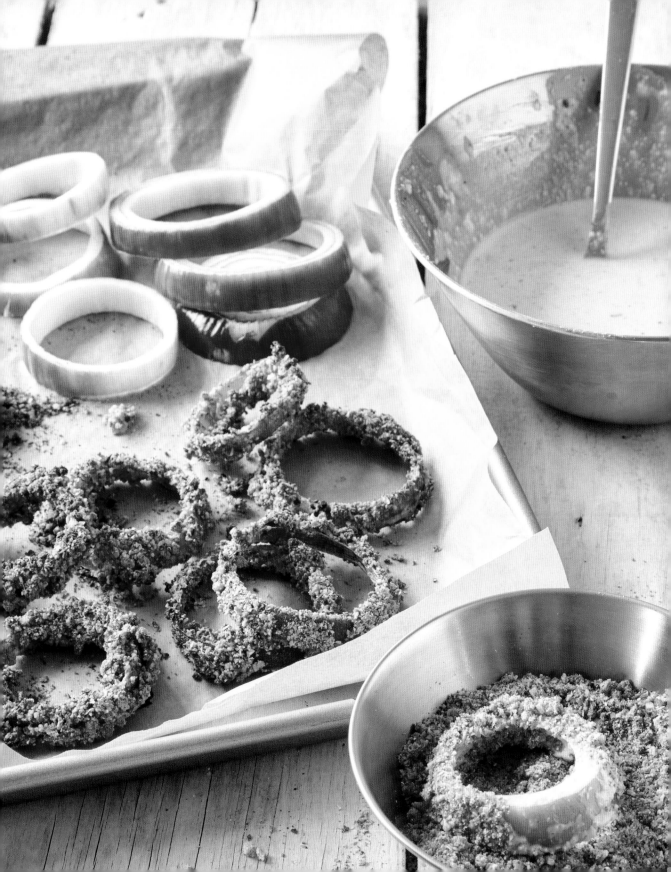

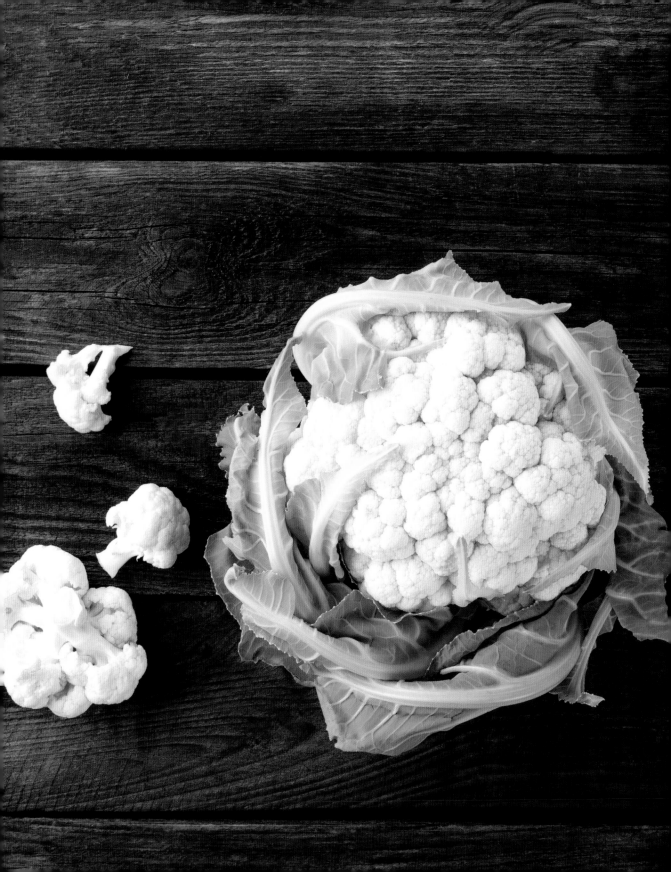

BUFFALO CAULIFLOWER WITH RANCH DRESSING

MAKES: *4* (1-CUP) SERVINGS · DIFFICULTY: *moderate*

This is a fun and delicious way to enjoy one of my favorite crucifers.

½ cup chickpea flour

1 tablespoon nutritional yeast

1 teaspoon garlic powder

1 teaspoon Savory Spice Blend (page 4)

1 head cauliflower, cut into bite-sized pieces

⅔ cup Healthy Hot Sauce (page 8)

Ranch Dressing (page 7)

Preheat the oven to 425°F. Line one or two large baking sheets with a silicone mat or parchment paper and set aside.

In a large bowl, combine the flour, nutritional yeast, garlic powder, and Savory Spice Blend. Stream in ½ cup of water and whisk until smooth. Add the cauliflower to the batter, turning to coat each piece. Arrange the battered cauliflower on the prepared baking sheets. (Do not let them touch.) Bake for 15 minutes, turning halfway through.

Pour the Healthy Hot Sauce in a large bowl. When the cauliflower is done, remove it from the oven and gently toss it in the hot sauce. Return the cauliflower pieces to the baking sheet. Bake for 20 to 25 minutes longer, or until they become crispy. Allow to cool for 10 minutes before serving with a side of Ranch Dressing.

Daily Dozen Foods

X BEANS　　X CRUCIFEROUS VEGETABLES　　X NUTS AND SEEDS　　X HERBS AND SPICES　　X WHOLE GRAINS

ELEVEN

SWEETS

You only need refined flour, sugar, eggs, and dairy to make sweet treats if you want desserts that will wreak havoc with your health. Using date sugar and date syrup as sweeteners, blending ground flaxseeds with warm water to replace eggs, and grinding old-fashioned oats into flour are just a few of the secrets to making delicious, decadent, whole-food desserts. For a quick sweet nibble, try the No-Bake Oatmeal Walnut Cookies. For a home-style dessert, dig into Baked Apple Crumbles, Two-Berry Pie with Pecan-Sunflower Crust, and Raspberry-Peach Crisp. Get your chocolate fix with Berry Chocolate Chia Pudding, Almond-Chocolate Truffles, and Fudgy No-Bake Brownies. What about a homemade soft-serve ice-cream-y type of dessert? It's as near as the frozen bananas in your freezer.

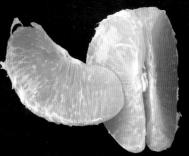

ALMOND-CHOCOLATE TRUFFLES

NO-BAKE OATMEAL WALNUT COOKIES

BAKED APPLE CRUMBLES

FRESH FRUIT SKEWERS WITH
BLACKBERRY COULIS

RASPBERRY-PEACH CRISP

STRAWBERRY-BANANA NICE CREAM

FUDGY NO-BAKE BROWNIES

BERRY CHOCOLATE CHIA PUDDING

TWO-BERRY PIE WITH
PECAN-SUNFLOWER CRUST

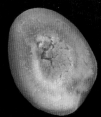

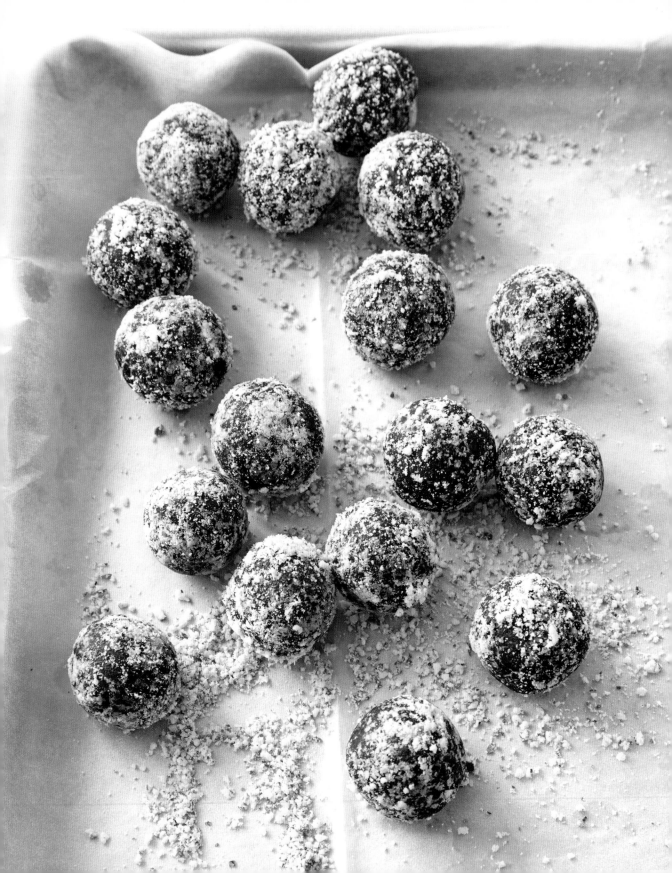

ALMOND-CHOCOLATE TRUFFLES

MAKES: ABOUT *24* · DIFFICULTY: *easy*

I've always had a sweet tooth, and the best way I can satisfy it is with fresh fruits like mangoes or dried fruits like dates. If you're going to have something sweet, you might as well make it something that's also nutritious.

⅓ cup chopped and pitted soft dates

⅓ cup raw cashews, soaked in hot water for 3 hours and then drained

3 tablespoons almond butter

½ cup unsweetened cocoa powder

¼ cup date sugar

1 2- to 3-inch piece vanilla bean, split and scraped (or 1 teaspoon extract)

Ground almonds, for coating

Combine the dates and cashews in a food processor and process to a paste. Add the almond butter and process to combine. Add the cocoa powder, date sugar, vanilla, and 1 teaspoon of water. Pulse until well combined.

Pinch some of the mixture between your fingers to see whether it holds together. If it's too dry, add a little more water, 1 teaspoon at a time, until the mixture can be shaped into balls. If the mixture is too soft, refrigerate it for 20 minutes or longer to firm up. If it's still too soft, add a little more cocoa powder, 1 teaspoon at a time.

Use your hands to shape and roll a small amount of the mixture into a 1-inch ball and transfer to a plate. Repeat until all the mixture has been rolled into balls.

Place the ground almonds in a shallow bowl. Roll the truffles in the almonds until they're coated, pressing on them if needed to cover completely. Transfer the coated truffles to a plate and refrigerate until firm before serving.

NOTE: If your dates are not soft, soak them in hot water for 20 minutes; then drain and pat dry before using.

Daily Dozen Foods

✗ **OTHER FRUITS**   ✗ **NUTS AND SEEDS**

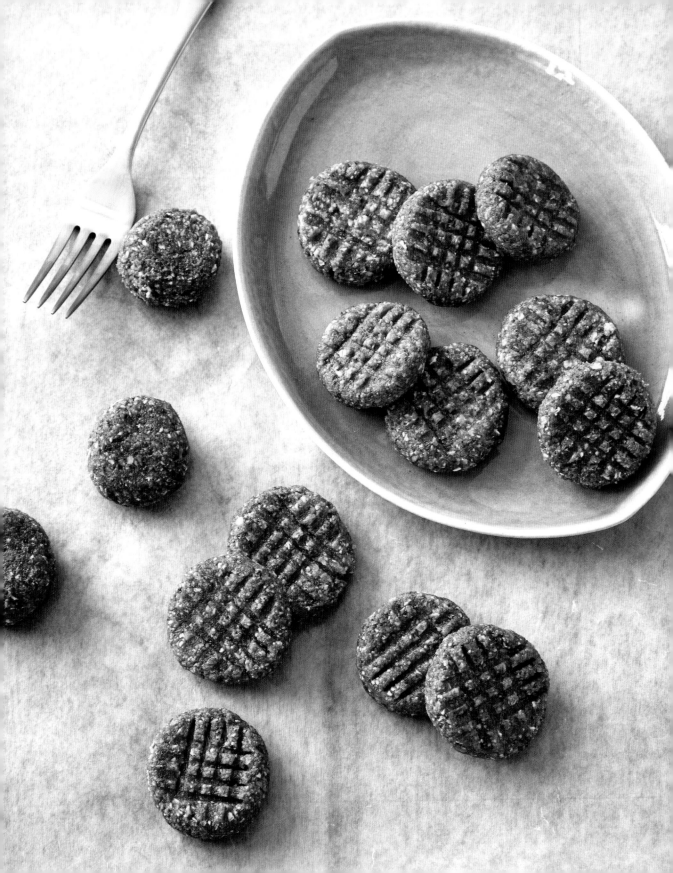

NO-BAKE OATMEAL
WALNUT COOKIES

MAKES: *24* COOKIES · DIFFICULTY: *easy*

These delicious treats can be assembled in minutes. Then simply pop them in the fridge to firm up before devouring.

1½ cups soft, pitted dates

1 cup walnut pieces

1 cup old-fashioned rolled oats

2 tablespoons date sugar, or to taste

1 tablespoon ground flaxseeds blended with 2 tablespoons warm water

1 2- to 3-inch piece vanilla bean, split and scraped (or 1 teaspoon extract)

1 teaspoon ground cinnamon

Line a baking sheet with a silicone mat or parchment paper and set aside. In a food processor, combine the dates, walnuts, and oats and process until crumbly. Add the date sugar, flax mixture, vanilla, and cinnamon and process until the dough holds together. If the mixture is too dry to hold together, add a little water, 1 tablespoon at a time. Scoop out about 1 tablespoon of the dough and roll it between your hands to form a ball. Repeat until all the dough is used. Arrange the balls on the prepared baking sheet, spaced liberally. Use a fork to press them down to flatten slightly and make a crisscross pattern. Refrigerate for 4 hours to firm up before serving.

Daily Dozen Foods

✗ OTHER FRUITS   ✗ FLAXSEEDS   ✗ NUTS AND SEEDS   ✗ HERBS AND SPICES   ✗ WHOLE GRAINS

BAKED APPLE CRUMBLES

MAKES: *4* SERVINGS · DIFFICULTY: *easy*

These baked apples have all the flavor (and wonderful fragrance) of apple pie, but are much better for you.

¼ cup finely chopped raw walnuts

¼ cup old-fashioned rolled oats

1 tablespoon raisins

1 tablespoon almond butter

1 teaspoon ground cinnamon

4 large firm baking apples, washed and cored

1 teaspoon blended peeled lemon (see page 3)

1 tablespoon Date Syrup (page 3)

Preheat the oven to 350°F. In a food processor, combine the walnuts, oats, raisins, almond butter, and cinnamon. Pulse until well mixed. Set the crumbled mixture aside.

Peel the apples about one-fourth down from the top. Rub the exposed part of the apples with the lemon to prevent discoloration. Stuff the crumble mixture into the center of the cored apples. Spoon the Date Syrup on top of the crumble mixture, dividing evenly. Arrange the apples upright in a shallow baking dish and pour ½ cup of water around them. Cover and bake until tender, about 1 hour. Serve warm.

VARIATION: If you want to save time, you can "bake" the apples in a microwave oven. Proceed as above; then arrange the apples in a microwave-safe baking dish. Microwave, uncovered, on high power until the apples are tender, 5 to 8 minutes, or longer, depending on the power of your microwave. Set aside to cool for 5 minutes before serving as the apples will be very hot inside.

APPLES

"An apple a day keeps the oncologist away." This was the title of a study published in the *Annals of Oncology* that set out to determine whether eating an apple (or more) a day was associated with lower cancer risk. The results: Compared with people who average less than one apple a day, daily apple eaters had 24 percent lower odds of breast cancer, as well as significantly lower risks for ovarian cancer, laryngeal cancer, and colorectal cancer.[135]

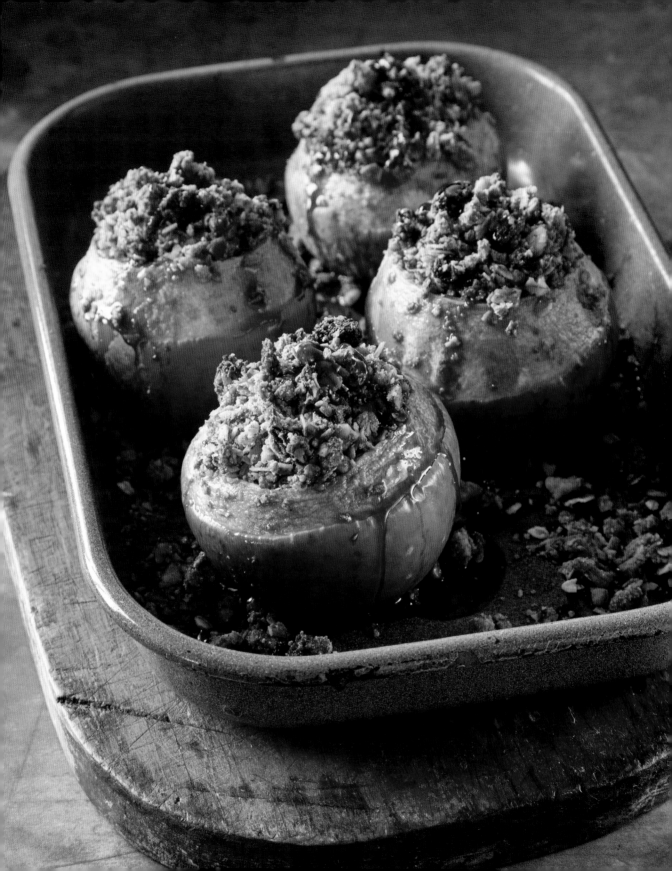

FRESH FRUIT SKEWERS WITH BLACKBERRY COULIS

MAKES: *4* SERVINGS · DIFFICULTY: *easy*

This is an easy, elegant, and fun way to enjoy fresh fruit. Mix and match the types of fruit depending on what's in season.

2 cups blackberries

½ teaspoon blended peeled lemon (see page 3)

Date sugar

1 cup hulled strawberries or raspberries

½ pineapple, peeled, cored, and cut into 1½-inch chunks

1 cup seedless red grapes

2 kiwi fruit, peeled and quartered

3 plums or peaches, halved, pitted, and cut into 1½-inch chunks

In a food processor or blender, combine the blackberries, lemon, and date sugar to taste, and process until smooth. Cover and refrigerate the coulis until needed.

Thread one piece of each type of fruit onto a skewer, adding additional fruit, depending on the length of your skewers. Arrange the skewered fruit on a platter and serve with the coulis, either drizzled on the fruit or served on the side in small bowls.

BERRIES

Berries aren't just one of the most important foods you can eat—they're also one of the most delicious. I buy big bags of them frozen so I never have to worry about whether or not they're in season. I even started growing them. The elderberry bush in our backyard is now taller than I am. The healthiest common fresh berries are probably blackberries, but I'm always on the lookout for local pick-your-own black raspberries.

Daily Dozen Foods

✗ BERRIES ✗ OTHER FRUITS

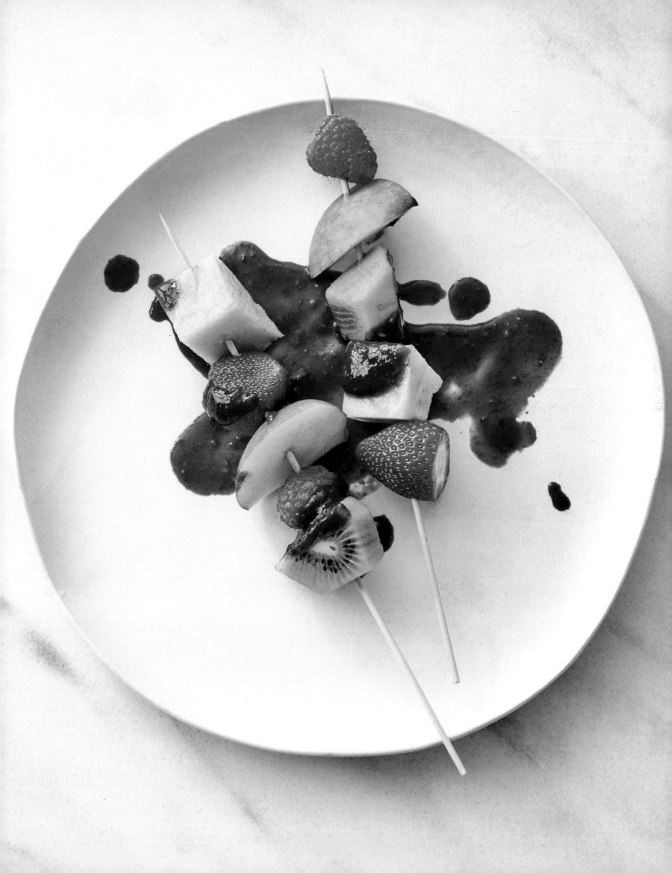

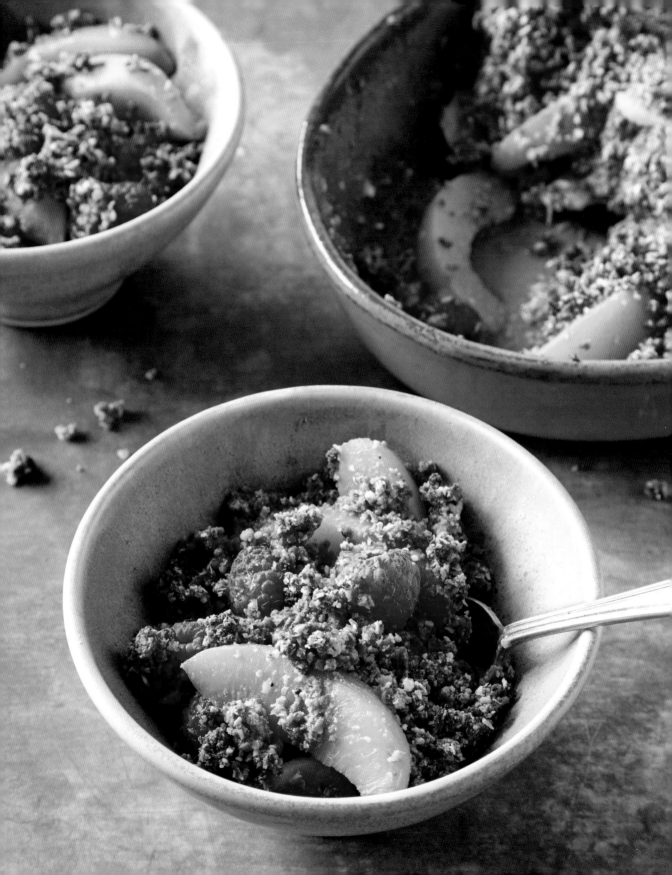

RASPBERRY-PEACH CRISP

MAKES: *6* (1-CUP) SERVINGS · DIFFICULTY: *easy*

I'm a fan of eating seasonally whenever I can. Why not change up the fruit in this recipe according to what's in season?

TOPPING

1 cup old-fashioned rolled oats

½ cup raw pecans

¼ cup pitted dates

¼ cup date sugar

½ teaspoon ground cinnamon

FILLING

¼ cup raw cashews, soaked in hot water for 3 hours, then drained

4 cups sliced peaches

⅓ cup date sugar, or more to taste

1 teaspoon blended peeled lemon (see page 3)

1 2- to 3-inch piece vanilla bean, split and scraped (or 1 teaspoon extract)

1½ cups raspberries

TOPPING: In a food processor, combine the oats, pecans, and dates, and pulse until finely ground. Add 2 tablespoons of water, date sugar, and cinnamon and pulse until the mixture is well combined and crumbly. Set aside. Preheat the oven to 350°F.

FILLING: In a high-speed blender, combine 2 tablespoons of water with the cashews, 1 cup of peach slices, date sugar, lemon, and vanilla and blend until smooth. In an 8-inch square baking pan or shallow baking dish, combine the remaining 3 cups of peaches with the raspberries. Pour the mixture from the blender over the fruit, mixing gently to combine and spread evenly.

Crumble the topping over the fruit. Bake for 25 to 30 minutes, or until the topping begins to brown and the filling is bubbling. Allow to cool for a few minutes before serving.

Daily Dozen Foods

✗ OTHER FRUITS   ✗ NUTS AND SEEDS   ✗ WHOLE GRAINS

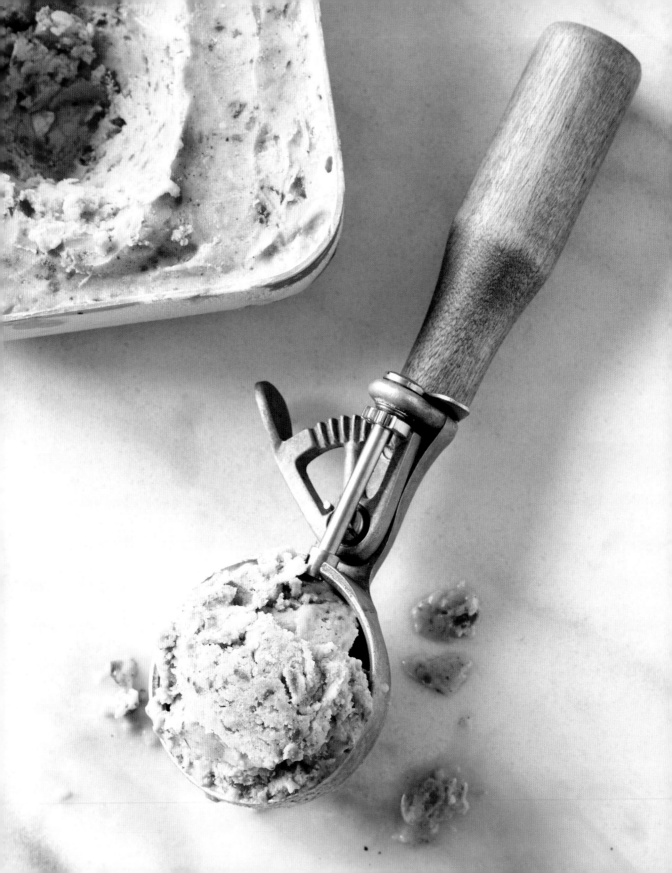

STRAWBERRY-BANANA NICE CREAM

MAKES: *4* (½-CUP) SERVINGS · DIFFICULTY: *easy*

I scream, you scream, we all scream for NICE cream! We can't get enough of this dessert in our household—both this specific recipe and easy-to-make, delicious variations. Here are four other favorites:

PEANUT BUTTER-BANANA: Omit the strawberries and use peanut butter instead of almond butter.

CHOCOLATEY BANANA: Instead of the strawberries, add cocoa powder for a healthy chocolate nice cream that tastes like a banana split.

VERY CHERRY: Replace the strawberries with fresh or frozen pitted cherries.

MATCHA: Simply blend two ingredients—powdered matcha green tea and blended frozen bananas—before freezing. (Please make sure the matcha is sourced from Japan, not China, due to lead contamination concerns.)

---

4 frozen overripe bananas, broken into chunks before freezing

2 tablespoons almond butter

1 cup sliced strawberries

1 1- to 1½-inch piece vanilla bean, split and scraped (or ½ teaspoon extract)

Combine the bananas and almond butter in a food processor and blend until smooth and creamy. Add the strawberries and vanilla and pulse to mix well, leaving a few solid bits of strawberry throughout. Transfer the nice cream to an airtight container and freeze for 30 minutes for a soft texture or for 1 to 2 hours for a firmer texture. If the nice cream becomes too hard to scoop, let it stand at room temperature for 10 to 15 minutes before serving.

TIP: Keep a stash of ripe banana chunks in the freezer to make delicious soft-serve nice cream (and smoothies) in minutes.

Daily Dozen Foods

X **BERRIES**   X **OTHER FRUITS**   X **NUTS AND SEEDS**

FUDGY NO-BAKE BROWNIES

MAKES: *16* (2-INCH) SQUARE BROWNIES · DIFFICULTY: *easy*

A quick and easy way to satisfy your sweet tooth while keeping it healthy.

1 cup walnuts

1⅓ cups dates, pitted

½ cup almond butter

½ cup unsweetened cocoa powder

⅓ cup crushed pecans

Grind the walnuts and dates in a food processor until finely ground. Add the almond butter and process until well mixed. Add the cocoa powder and pulse to mix well.

Transfer the brownie mixture to an 8-inch square baking pan. (If you line the pan with parchment paper, it will make it easier to remove the brownies.) Use your fingers to press the mixture evenly into the pan. (You can place a piece of parchment paper on top of the mixture as you press it into the pan to prevent it from sticking to your hands.) Once the brownies are firmly pressed into the pan, sprinkle the top evenly with the crushed pecans, pressing them into the top of the brownies. Cover and refrigerate for at least 1 hour before cutting into squares.

Daily Dozen Foods

✗ OTHER FRUITS   ✗ NUTS AND SEEDS

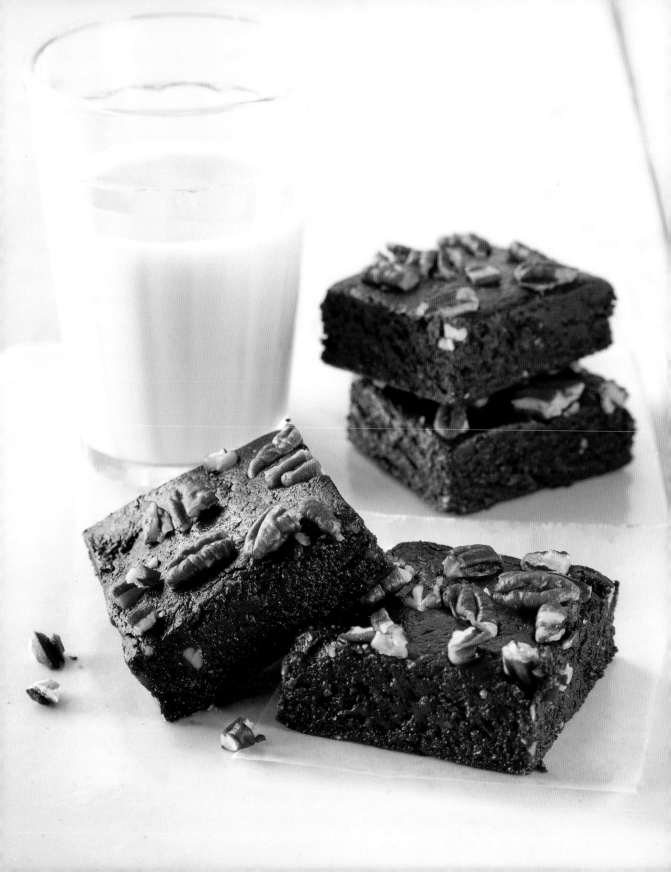

BERRY CHOCOLATE CHIA PUDDING

MAKES: *4* (¾-CUP) SERVINGS · DIFFICULTY: *easy*

Avocado and almond butter add richness to this chocolaty pudding.

½ ripe Hass avocado, halved and pitted

1¼ cups strawberries, blueberries, or other berries of choice

3 tablespoons unsweetened cacao powder

2 tablespoons almond butter

½ cup Date Syrup (page 3)

1½ cups Almond Milk (page 2)

¼ cup chia seeds

Optional garnishes: fresh berries, raw slivered almonds, cacao nibs

Scoop out the flesh from the avocado and place it in a high-speed blender or food processor. Add the berries, cacao powder, almond butter, Date Syrup, and Almond Milk. Blend until completely smooth and then pour into a bowl. Whisk in the chia seeds until they're evenly distributed. Cover and refrigerate for at least 8 hours. Divide the pudding among four small dessert bowls, garnish as desired, and refrigerate for 20 minutes before serving.

Daily Dozen Foods

✗ BERRIES   ✗ OTHER FRUITS   ✗ NUTS AND SEEDS

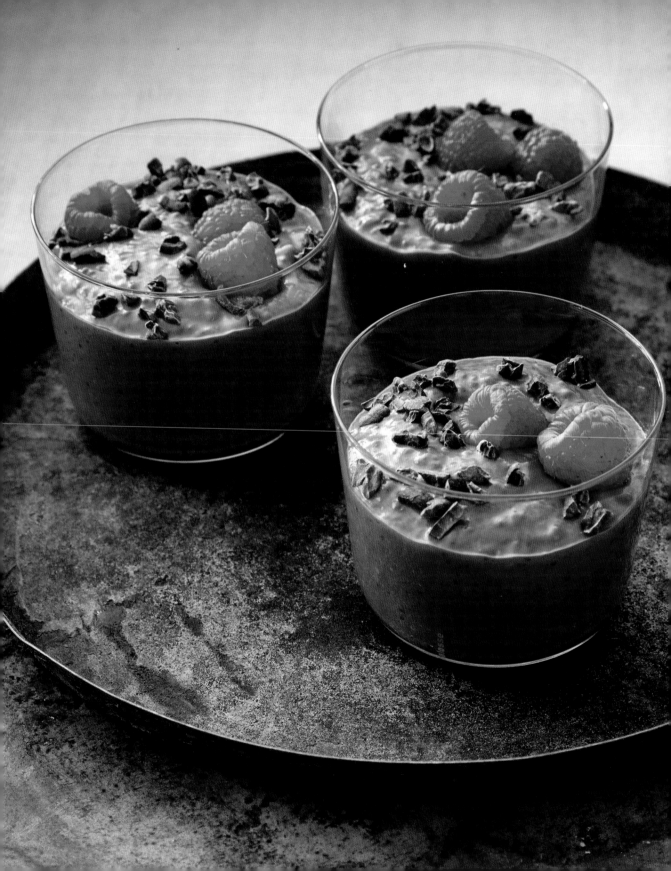

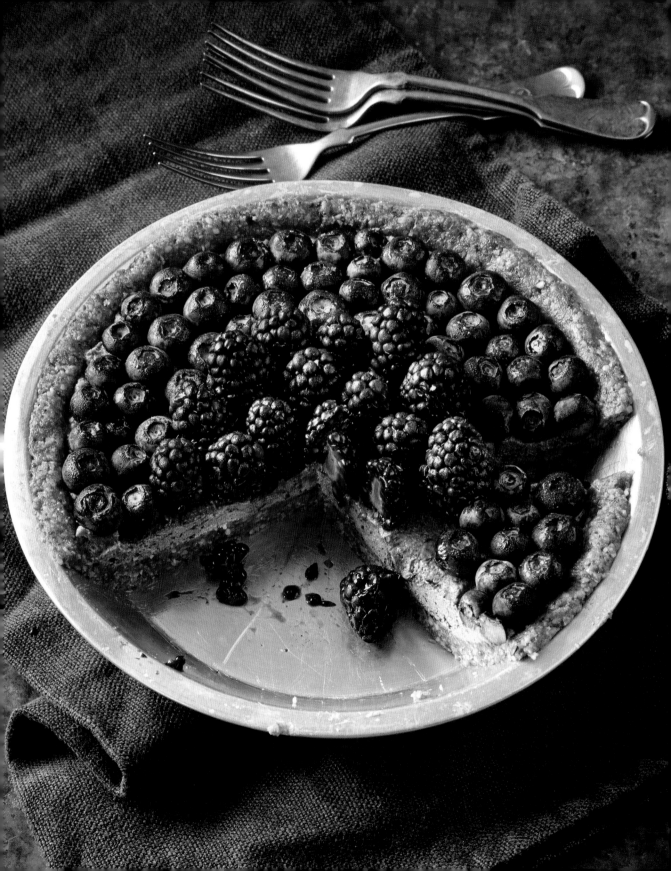

TWO-BERRY PIE WITH PECAN-SUNFLOWER CRUST

MAKES: *8* SERVINGS • DIFFICULTY: *easy*

An easy, three-ingredient crust is the base for this delicious pie with a creamy layer of filling and a fresh berry topping.

CRUST

1 cup pecans or walnuts

¾ cup sunflower seeds

½ cup soft, pitted Medjool dates

FILLING

¾ cup cashews, soaked for 3 hours in hot water, then drained

2 tablespoons date sugar

½ teaspoon blended peeled lemon (see page 3)

1 1- to 1½-inch piece vanilla bean, split and scraped (or ½ teaspoon extract)

½ ripe banana

1¼ cups fresh blueberries, or thawed frozen

1 cup fresh blackberries or small strawberries, or thawed frozen

CRUST: Combine all three of the crust ingredients in a food processor and process until coarsely ground. If the mixture doesn't hold together when pinched, add 1 to 2 tablespoons of water. Press the crust mixture into a 9-inch pie plate (lined with plastic wrap for easy removal, if desired) or springform pan and set aside. Refrigerate the crust while you prepare the filling.

FILLING: Blend the drained cashews, date sugar, lemon, and vanilla in a high-speed blender and blend until smooth. Add the banana and ½ cup of the blueberries, and blend until smooth and creamy. Spread the filling evenly on top of the crust.

Arrange the blackberries and remaining ¾ cup of blueberries in concentric circles on top of the filling. Refrigerate for 4 hours to firm up before serving. For best results, serve this pie on the same day it is made.

Daily Dozen Foods

✗ BERRIES   ✗ OTHER FRUITS   ✗ NUTS AND SEEDS

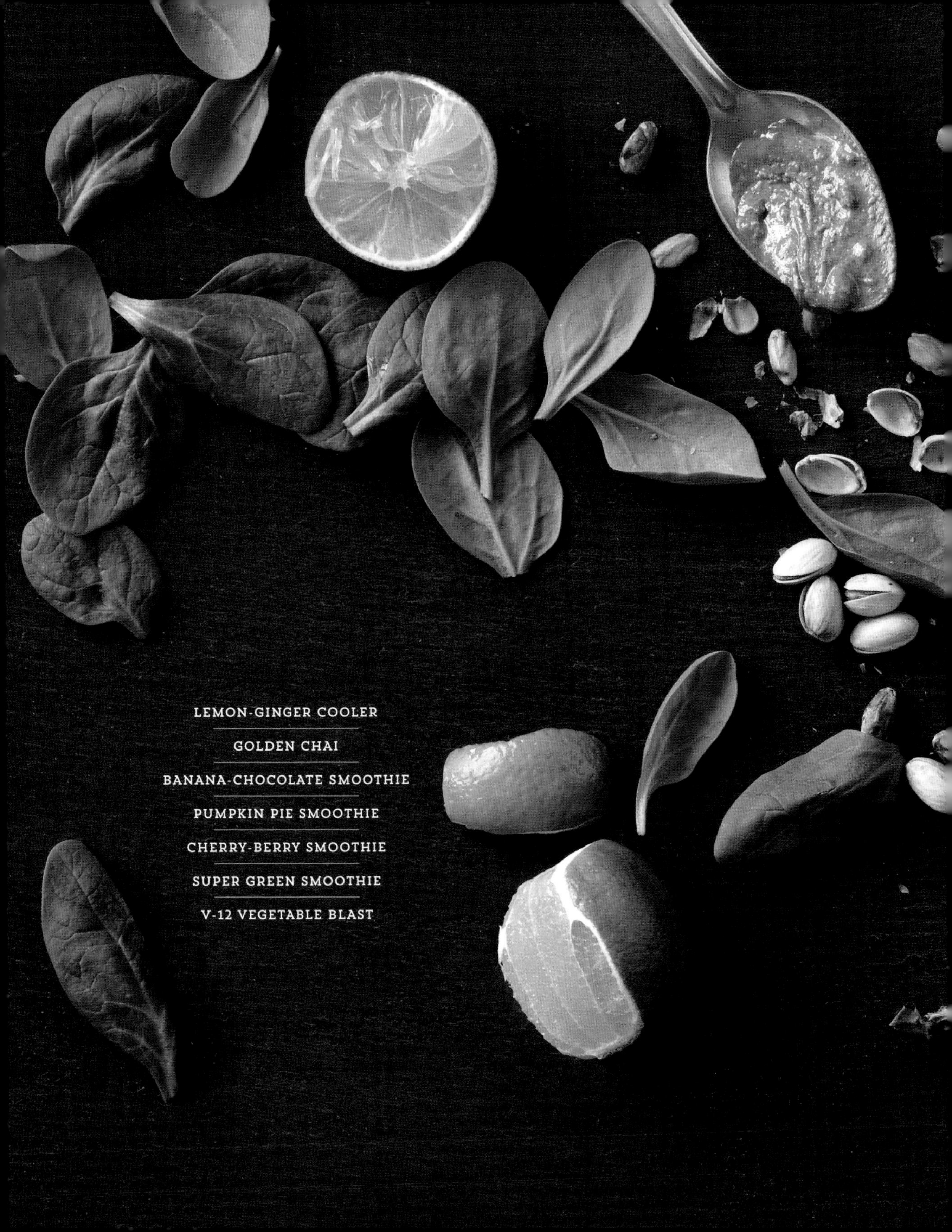

LEMON-GINGER COOLER

GOLDEN CHAI

BANANA-CHOCOLATE SMOOTHIE

PUMPKIN PIE SMOOTHIE

CHERRY-BERRY SMOOTHIE

SUPER GREEN SMOOTHIE

V-12 VEGETABLE BLAST

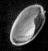

SIPS

Smoothie fans will enjoy the selection we've put together, ranging from Super Green to a decadent-tasting Banana-Chocolate. The Cherry-Berry Smoothie tastes like summer, and the Pumpkin Pie Smoothie is perfect for the fall and winter. If I had to pick just one, my favorite new concoction is the V-12 Vegetable Blast.

LEMON-GINGER COOLER

MAKES: *2* (2-CUP) SERVINGS • DIFFICULTY: *easy*

You can also serve this scintillating beverage as a hot tea.

---

1 2-inch piece fresh ginger, sliced

2 tablespoons blended peeled lemon (see page 3)

1 4-inch piece cinnamon stick (optional)

Date Syrup (page 3) (optional)

Mint sprigs, for serving (optional)

Combine 4 cups of water with the ginger in a large saucepan and bring to a boil. Remove from the heat. Add the lemon and cinnamon stick (if using) and set aside for 30 minutes. Sweeten to taste with Date Syrup (if using). Refrigerate until chilled. Serve in tall glasses over ice. Add a sprig of mint if you're in the mood.

5 WAYS TO PEP UP YOUR WATER

Add any of the following to a glass or pitcher of water to make a good thing even better:

1. Lemon or lime slices
2. Cucumber slices
3. Ginger slices
4. Mint leaves
5. Ice cubes with fresh berries frozen inside

Daily Dozen Foods

✗ OTHER FRUITS   ✗ HERBS AND SPICES   ✗ BEVERAGES

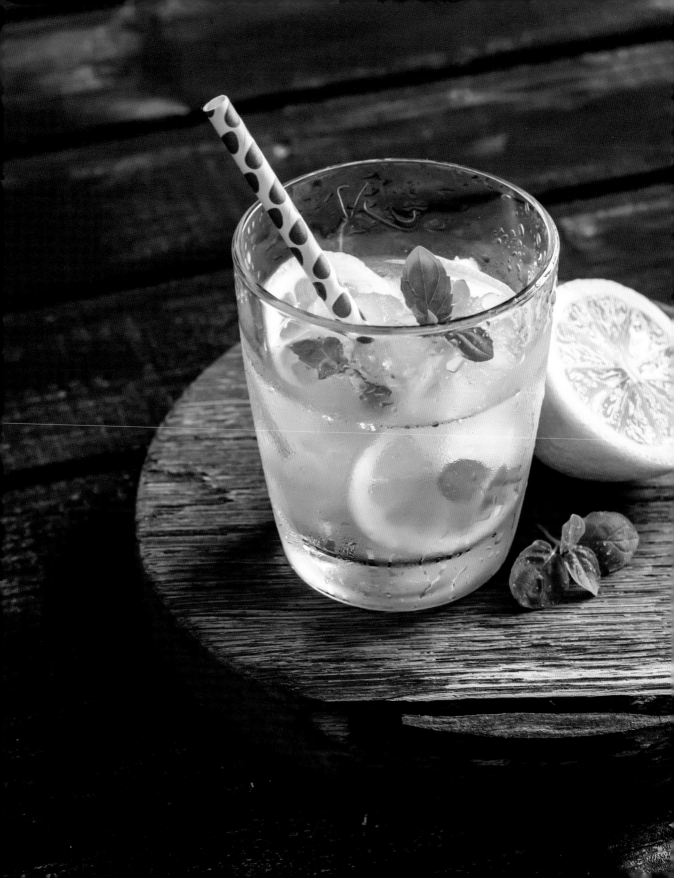

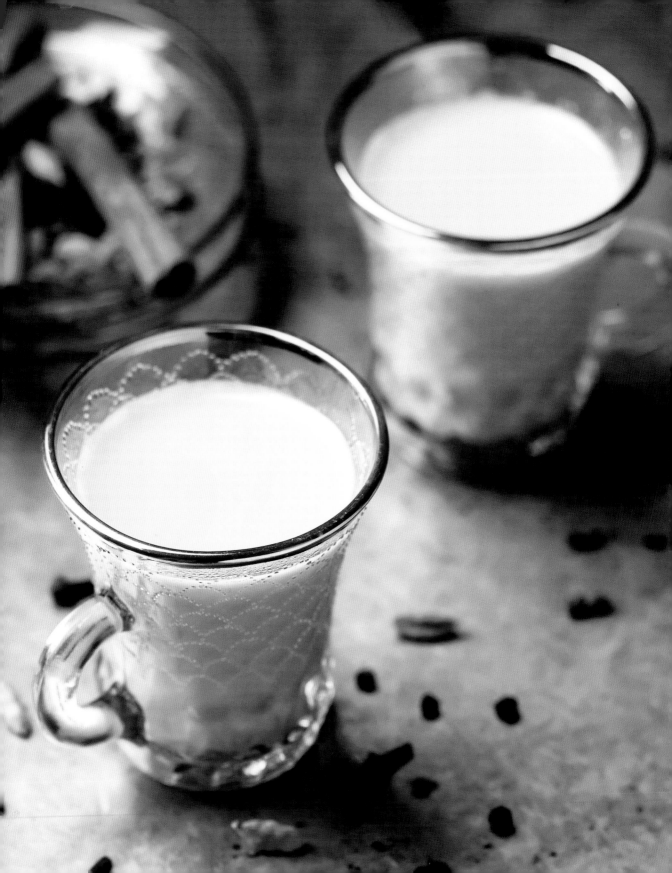

GOLDEN CHAI

MAKES: *4* (1¼-CUP) SERVINGS · DIFFICULTY: *easy*

Turmeric adds a touch of gold to this fragrant tea that can be served hot or cold.

2 2-inch pieces cinnamon stick

1 1-inch piece fresh ginger, cut into thin rounds

8 whole cloves

4 green cardamom pods, smashed

2 teaspoons fennel seeds

1 ¼-inch piece fresh turmeric, grated (or ¼ teaspoon ground)

6 cups cold water

6 bags Darjeeling or other black tea

¼ cup Date Syrup (page 3), or to taste

1 cup Almond Milk (page 2), or to taste

In a medium saucepan, combine the cinnamon, ginger, cloves, cardamom, fennel seeds, and turmeric. Add the water and bring to a boil. Reduce the heat to low and simmer for 10 minutes. Remove from the heat. Add the tea bags and steep for 5 minutes. Remove and discard the tea bags. Stir in the Date Syrup and Almond Milk. Strain the chai into a teapot and serve.

Daily Dozen Foods

X OTHER FRUITS   X NUTS AND SEEDS   X HERBS AND SPICES   X BEVERAGES

BANANA-CHOCOLATE SMOOTHIE

MAKES: *1* (2-CUP) SERVING · DIFFICULTY: *easy*

This creamy, chocolaty smoothie tastes so rich and delicious, you'll forget how healthy it is!

---

1 frozen ripe banana, cut into chunks before freezing

⅓ cup frozen blueberries

2 tablespoons unsweetened cocoa powder

1 tablespoon ground flaxseeds

1 1- to 1½-inch piece vanilla bean, split and scraped (or ½ teaspoon extract)

1 tablespoon almond butter

2 tablespoons Date Syrup (page 3) (optional, depending on the sweetness of the fruit)

1 cup raw spinach leaves

3 to 4 ice cubes (optional)

Combine all the ingredients with 1 cup of water in a high-speed blender. Blend until thick and smooth. For a thinner texture, add less ice (if using) or more water. Serve immediately.

SMOOTHIES

My smoothie strategy is to combine super-tasty foods with those that are less tasty, such as mangoes with raw kale, so they balance each other out. Smoothies let you consume foods you might not otherwise pack into your daily diet, and they're convenient. For me, this means I can be at my treadmill desk, exercising, working, and getting some of my Daily Dozen through a straw, all at the same time!

Some people have said that when you put veggies and fruit into a blender, the fiber is somehow lost. That's ridiculous. As much fiber as goes into the blender, comes out of the blender. What a good blender can do is break down fruit and vegetable cell walls better than our teeth, and this helps release more nutrition than we would get otherwise. To avoid feeling hungry after a smoothie, though, sip smoothies slowly so that your mind and body have time to register the intake and send appropriate fullness signals.

Daily Dozen Foods

X BERRIES   X OTHER FRUITS   X GREENS   X FLAXSEEDS   X NUTS AND SEEDS   X BEVERAGES

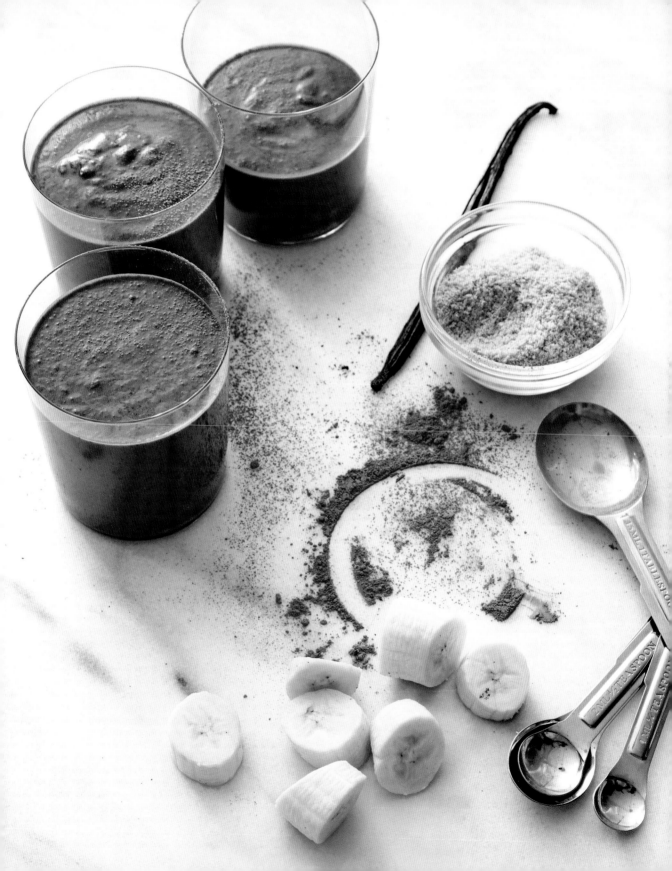

PUMPKIN PIE SMOOTHIE

MAKES: *1* (1¾-CUP) SERVING · DIFFICULTY: *easy*

This drink tastes just like pumpkin pie in a glass. Make sure you use solid-pack pure pumpkin purée and not pumpkin pie filling.

½ cup solid-pack pure pumpkin

1 small frozen ripe banana, cut into chunks before freezing

3 soft Medjool dates, pitted

1 ¼-inch piece fresh turmeric, grated (or ¼ teaspoon ground)

1 teaspoon pumpkin pie spice

1 tablespoon almond butter

Combine all the ingredients with 1 cup of water in a high-speed blender and blend until smooth. Serve immediately.

Daily Dozen Foods

✗ OTHER FRUITS   ✗ OTHER VEGETABLES   ✗ NUTS AND SEEDS   ✗ BEVERAGES

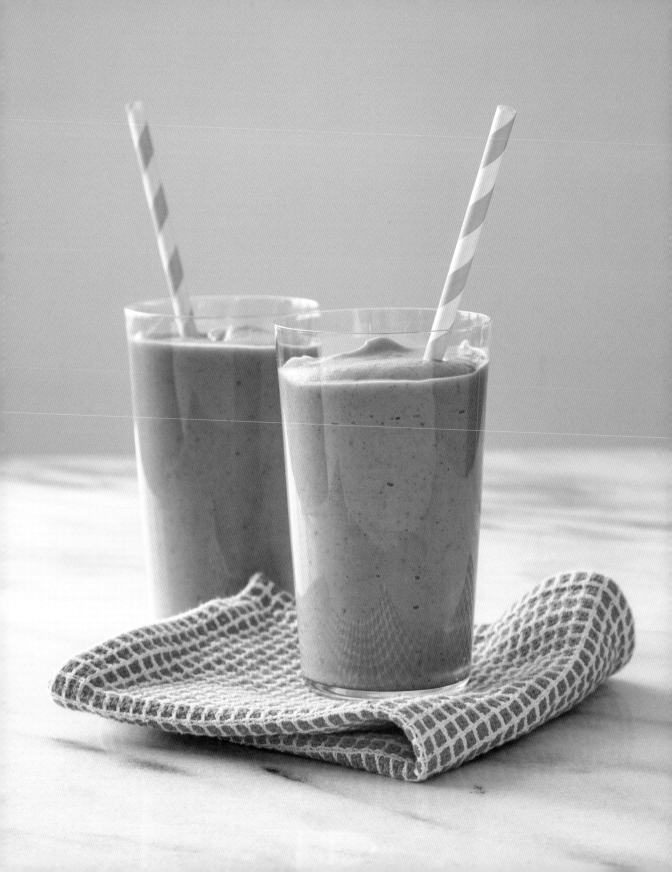

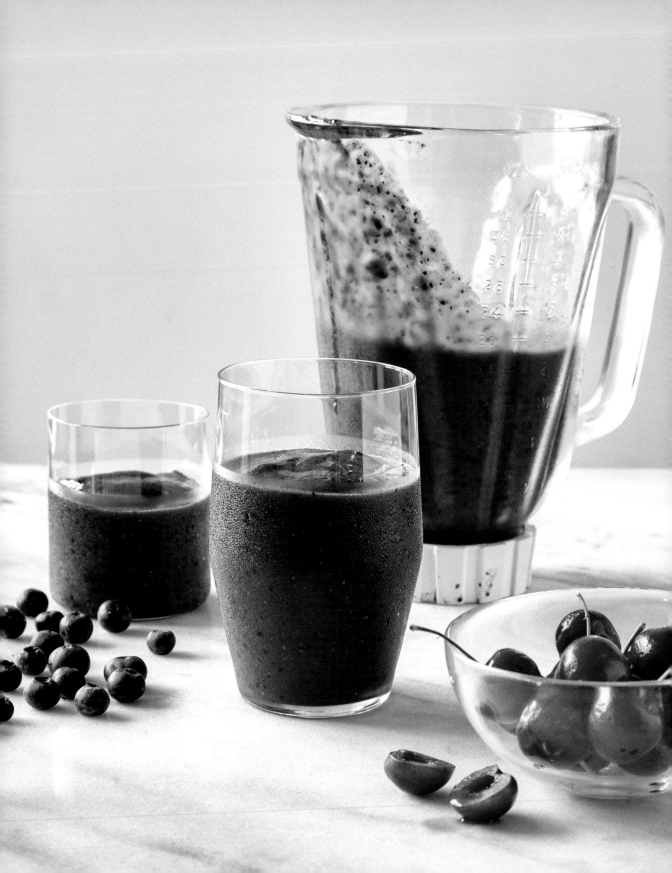

CHERRY-BERRY SMOOTHIE

MAKES: *1* (2½-CUP) SERVING · DIFFICULTY: *easy*

This is a great go-to smoothie that can be enjoyed year-round if you keep some berries stashed in the freezer. Mix and match the types of berries (or use other fresh or frozen fruit) to change things up. If your fruit isn't sweet enough, add a soft date or two or a drizzle of Date Syrup (page 3) to taste.

1 cup frozen blueberries

½ cup fresh or frozen pitted cherries

1 frozen ripe banana, cut into chunks before freezing

1 tablespoon ground flaxseeds

1 tablespoon almond butter

Combine all the ingredients with 1½ cups of water in a blender and blend until smooth and creamy, about 1 minute. Add more water if you prefer a thinner consistency. Serve immediately.

Daily Dozen Foods

✗ BERRIES   ✗ OTHER FRUITS   ✗ FLAXSEEDS   ✗ NUTS AND SEEDS   ✗ BEVERAGES

SUPER GREEN SMOOTHIE

MAKES: *1* (2½-CUP) SERVING · DIFFICULTY: *easy*

You can check off six of the Daily Dozen scorecard boxes with this delicious and refreshing drink. Six with just one smoothie! For a thinner texture, add a little more water, if desired.

2 cups packed fresh baby spinach

1 large apple, cored

1 cup diced pineapple

½ ripe Hass avocado, peeled and pitted

¼ cup packed fresh mint leaves

3 soft Medjool dates, pitted

1 ¼-inch piece fresh turmeric, grated (or ¼ teaspoon ground)

2 teaspoons blended peeled lemon or lime (see page 3)

1 tablespoon ground flaxseeds

Ice cubes (optional)

In a blender, combine all the ingredients and blend until completely smooth. Add ⅔ cup or more of water and ice (if using) and blend until smooth. Serve immediately.

Daily Dozen Foods

✗ OTHER FRUITS   ✗ GREENS   ✗ OTHER VEGETABLES   ✗ NUTS AND SEEDS   ✗ HERBS AND SPICES   ✗ BEVERAGES

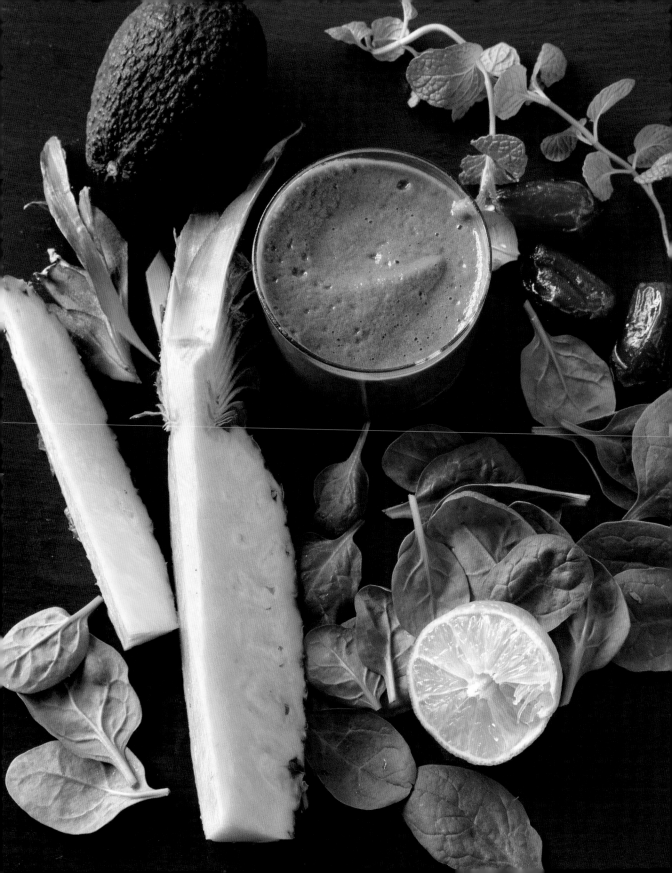

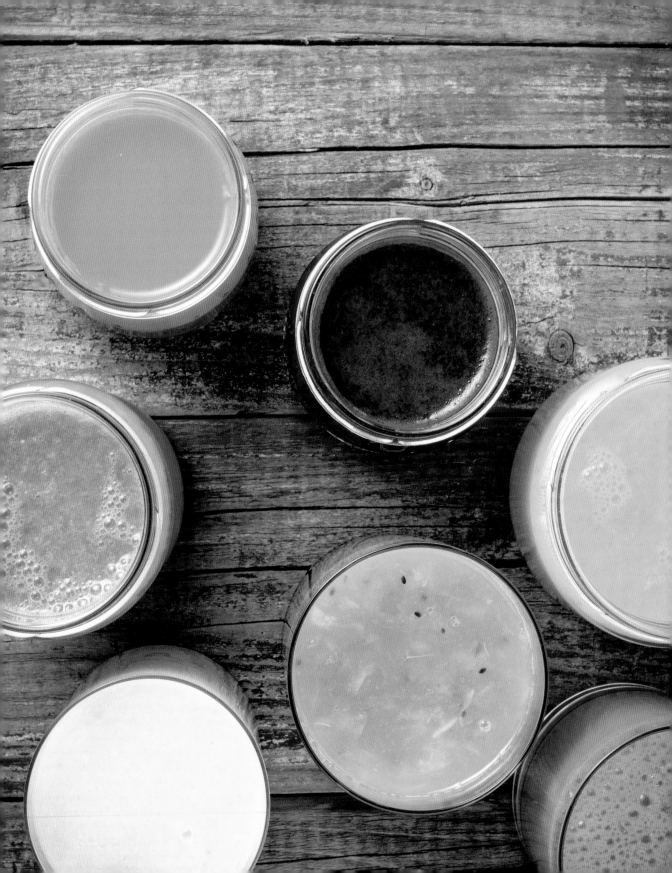

V-12 VEGETABLE BLAST

MAKES: *2* (12-OUNCE) SERVINGS · DIFFICULTY: *easy*

This is a great way to drink your vegetables!

---

2 cups spinach, red kale, or other dark greens

1 or 2 plum tomatoes

1 celery rib, coarsely chopped

½ red bell pepper, quartered

1 tablespoon chopped red onion, or 1 small garlic clove

½ jalapeño pepper, seeded (optional, but whoo-hoo!)

2 teaspoons blended peeled lemon (see page 3)

1 apple, cored and quartered

2 teaspoons chlorella (optional)

1 ¼-inch piece fresh turmeric, grated (or ¼ teaspoon ground)

½ cup ice cubes

Combine all the ingredients with 2 cups of water in a high-speed blender and blend until smooth. Transfer to large glasses and serve.

Daily Dozen Foods

✗ OTHER FRUITS   ✗ GREENS   ✗ OTHER VEGETABLES   ✗ HERBS AND SPICES   ✗ BEVERAGES

PEOPLE OFTEN ASK ME FOR MORE THAN RECIPES

They want suggestions on how to create meal plans for a week or more. To honor those requests, here are two full weeks of menu preparations. You can also check out my Lighter profile for free meal plans incorporating hundreds of recipes at www.lighter.world/providers/Michael_Greger

WEEK 1

DAY 1

BREAKFAST
Summertime Oatmeal

LUNCH
Curried Chickpea Wraps
V-12 Vegetable Blast

DINNER
Super Salad with Garlic Caesar Dressing
& Hemp Hearts
Zucchini Noodles with Avocado-Cashew Alfredo

DESSERT
Strawberry-Banana Nice Cream

DAY 2

BREAKFAST
Burrito Breakfast Bake

LUNCH
Vegetable & Red Bean Gumbo
Cheesy Kale Crisps

DINNER
Miso Soup with Spinach & Dulse
Buckwheat Soba & Edamame
with Almond Butter Sauce

DESSERT
Berry Chocolate Chia Pudding

DAY 3

BREAKFAST
Morning Grain Bowls

LUNCH
Spinach & Mushroom Black Bean Burritos
Edamame Guacamole + raw veggies

DINNER
Mango-Avocado-Kale Salad with
Ginger-Sesame Orange Dressing
Yellow Rice & Black Beans with Broccoli

DESSERT
Fudgy No-Bake Brownies

DAY 4

BREAKFAST
Super Green Smoothie

LUNCH
Black Bean Gazpacho Salad
Pumpkin Seed Dip + raw veggies

DINNER
Stuffed Portobellos with Herbed Mushroom Gravy
Purple Cabbage Sauté

DESSERT
Baked Apple Crumbles

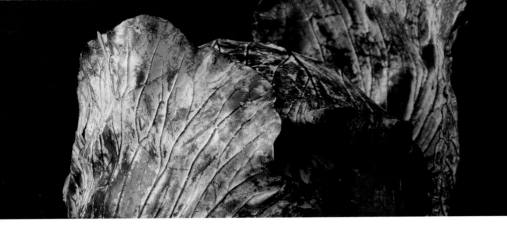

DAY 5

BREAKFAST
French Toast with Berry Drizzle
Warm Pear Compote

LUNCH
Kale & White Bean Soup
Three-Seed Crackers

DINNER
Super Salad with Garlic Caesar Dressing
& Hemp Hearts
Roasted Vegetable Lasagna

DESSERT
Very Cherry Nice Cream

DAY 6

BREAKFAST
Skillet Sweet Potato Hash
100% whole-grain toast

LUNCH
Beans & Greens Quesadillas
Summer Salsa

DINNER
Portobellos & Greens on Toast
Baked Onion Rings

DESSERT
Two-Berry Pie with Pecan-Sunflower Crust

DAY 7

BREAKFAST
French Toast with Berry Drizzle

LUNCH
Sloppy Jacks

DINNER
Lentil Shepherd's Pie
Roasted Asparagus with Yellow Pepper Béarnaise

DESSERT
Almond-Chocolate Truffles

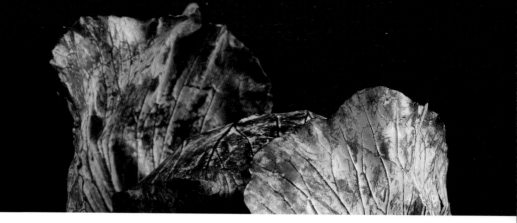

WEEK 2

DAY 8

BREAKFAST
Summertime Oatmeal

LUNCH
Moroccan Lentil Soup
Cheesy Kale Crisps

DINNER
Garlic Greens Sauté
Mac & Cheese

DESSERT
Raspberry-Peach Crisp

DAY 9

BREAKFAST
Pumpkin Pie Smoothie
Superfood Breakfast Bites

LUNCH
Chopped Vegetable Salad
Champion Vegetable Chili

DINNER
Quinoa Pilaf with Carrots & Chickpeas
Cauliflower Steaks with Chermoula Sauce

DESSERT
Strawberry-Banana Nice Cream

DAY 10

BREAKFAST
Chocolate Oatmeal

LUNCH
Black Bean Soup with Quinoa & Kale
Beet Burgers

DINNER
Pistachio-Spinach Salad with
Strawberry Balsamic Dressing
Whole Wheat Pasta with Lentil Bolognese

DESSERT
Fresh Fruit Skewers with Blackberry Coulis

DAY 11

BREAKFAST
Burrito Breakfast Bake

LUNCH
Smoky Black-Eyed Peas & Collards
Brown rice

DINNER
Chickpea & Cauliflower Curry
Brown rice
Indian-Style Spinach & Tomatoes

DESSERT
Fudgy No-Bake Brownies

DAY 12

BREAKFAST

Superfood Breakfast Bites

Cherry-Berry Smoothie

LUNCH

Veracruz Tempeh Lettuce Wraps

Smoky Roasted Chickpeas

DINNER

Braised Tempeh & Bok Choy
with Spicy Ginger Sauce

Brown rice

DESSERT

No-Bake Oatmeal Walnut Cookies

DAY 13

BREAKFAST

Morning Grain Bowls

LUNCH

Black Bean Burgers

Sesame Purple Cabbage & Carrot Slaw

DINNER

Roasted Beets with Balsamic-Braised Beet Greens

Stuffed Winter Squash with Black Bean Sauce

DESSERT

Peanut Butter–Banana Nice Cream

DAY 14

BREAKFAST

Skillet Sweet Potato Hash

100% whole-grain toast

LUNCH

Kale Salad with Avocado Goddess Dressing

Beans & Greens Quesadillas

DINNER

Lemon-Roasted Brussels Sprouts
& Carrots with Pecans

Red Quinoa Loaf with Golden Gravy

DESSERT

Fresh Fruit Skewers with Blackberry Coulis

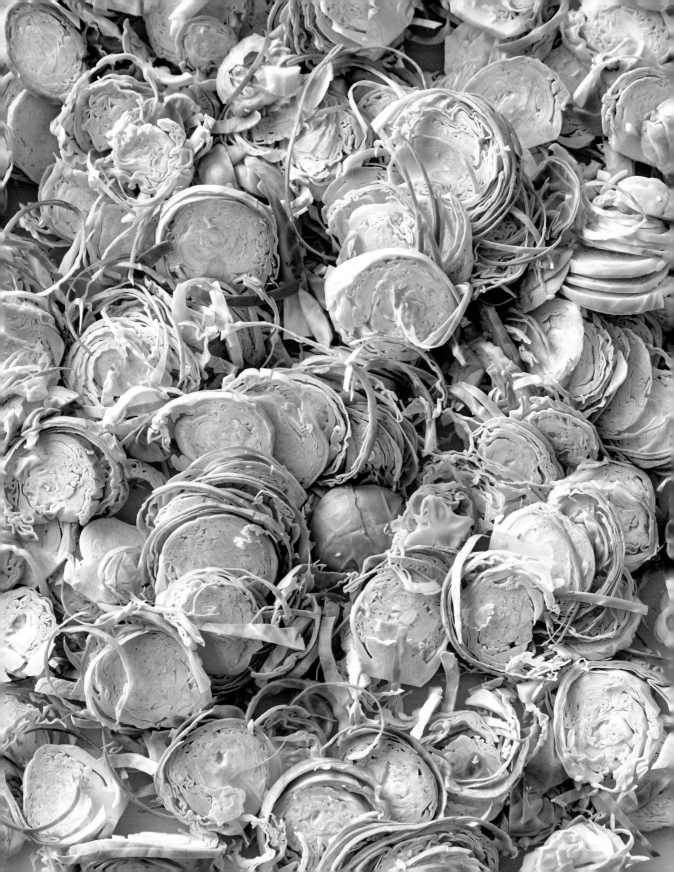

KITCHEN TECHNIQUES

Here's a handful of hints and explanations to help you in the kitchen:

BAKING: This dry-heat cooking method takes place in an oven, usually with a temperature below 400°F, primarily involving foods that lack structure before becoming solid, such as muffins or cakes.

BAKING AND ROASTING WITH SILICONE MATS OR PARCHMENT PAPER: Lining your baking sheets and pans with silicone mats or parchment paper before placing ingredients on them allows you to bake and roast without oil and without the food sticking. It also makes cleanup that much easier.

BRAISING: This cooking method uses both moist and dry heats. Typically, the food is first seared at a high temperature before being finished in a covered pot at a lower temperature with some cooking liquid that may also add flavor. The cooking liquid is then sometimes thickened to create a sauce or gravy.

ROASTING: Similar to baking, this dry-heat cooking method takes place in an oven, usually with a temperature at or above 400°F. Roasting involves cooking foods that already have a solid structure before the cooking process begins, such as vegetables.

SIMMERING: This is a technique in which foods are cooked in a hot liquid that is kept just below the boiling point of water. To keep a liquid simmering, bring it to a boil and then lower the heat to a point where the bubbles almost stop forming. Simmering is a gentle cooking method often used to cook soup and stews.

SOAKING AND BLENDING NUTS: Some recipes require nuts to be ground into sauces, nut milk, or nut cream. Compared with blanched almonds, cashews are softer and will grind more easily into a fine powder. In order to make the smoothest sauce possible, either first grind the nuts into a powder and blend the sauce long enough to achieve a smooth sauce or soak the nuts in water overnight or in hot water for a couple of hours.

STEAMING TEMPEH: Before using tempeh in recipes, it is advisable to steam it over simmering water for 15 to 30 minutes to help mellow its flavor.

STEAMING VEGETABLES: To steam vegetables, bring a few inches of water to a boil in a large saucepan. Arrange the vegetables in a steaming basket and set it over the boiling water, making sure that the vegetables aren't immersed in the water. Cover and let the vegetables steam until they're cooked to the desired tenderness. Check the water level, if needed, to be sure it doesn't all evaporate.

STIR-FRYING: This method of quick cooking over medium-high heat helps maintain the color, flavor, and texture of the foods you prepare. When you stir-fry, it's best to have your ingredients prepped and ready to go so they can be quickly tossed into the wok or pan. Different ingredients are added separately to a stir-fry. according to their different cooking times—for example thinly sliced mushrooms stir-fry in a few minutes, whereas diced carrots take longer. Once the ingredients are nearly cooked, add spices or a sauce and stir to coat the ingredients. Although stir-frying in oil is a common method, you can—and should—stir-fry in water instead for a healthier dish without the added empty calories.

WATER-SAUTÉING: This method is a way to sauté ingredients without using oil. To water-sauté, heat 2 tablespoons (or more, depending on the recipe) of water in a skillet over medium heat. Add your ingredients to the hot liquid and cook, stirring or turning as needed, until the ingredients have softened. In place of water, you can also sauté in wine, vinegar, Vegetable Broth (page 6), and even the liquid from a can of unsalted beans.

SHOPPING AND STOCKING THE PANTRY

I wrote this cookbook because people wanted recipes that would help them understand how to apply the principles in *How Not to Die* in their daily diet and to give them handy, delicious ways to get the Daily Dozen and other wonderful Green Light foods into their meals.

That's great if you're already committed to the most healthful way of eating. But I also wrote this book for those of you who may be at the experimental stage, where you are telling yourself, "Okay, I'm willing to try eating more healthfully, but I'm only going to do it if I like what's on my plate!"

To eat well, it helps to cook well, and to cook well, you need to have the right foods at the ready. And all that starts with shopping.

When I go to the grocery store, I am thinking mainly about three things: produce, produce, and produce. I try to stock the fridge with as many fresh vegetables and fruits as will fit.

A shopping spree in our household means spending almost all of our time in the produce aisle. I love seeing what new items are in season—such as peaches in the summer and squash in the winter. I try to make sure my cart mimics a rainbow. Besides all shades of greens, I might buy purple cabbage, yellow peppers, red apples, and blueberries. More colors mean the most plant pigments, which mean more antioxidants.

As part of our produce-gathering mission, I also spend time in the opposite side of the store, the frozen foods section. Sometimes frozen fruits and veggies actually contain more nutrition than fresh ones. Frozen vegetables may be frozen on the day of picking, whereas "fresh" produce may have been sitting on a ship from the other side of the Earth, losing some of its nutritional value along the way. Local and fresh-picked is best, but not available year-round where I live, which is why I hang out in the frozen foods aisle.

The only times I really fan out into the heart of the store is to buy whole-grain pastas, jarred or Tetra Pak tomato products, canned beans when I'm not cooking my own, and whole grains, dried beans, nuts and seeds, dried fruit, and spices from the bulk aisle. I like to make big batches of beans and greens so I have them always at the ready to instantly improve the nutrition of any dish. I hate to see good food go bad, so it provides that extra motivation to pack in the healthiest of foods.

As well, I keep lots of old bottles and shakers sitting out on the kitchen island. I keep them brimming with spice mixes I've created, chia seeds, pumpkin seeds, dried parsley, dried peppermint, dried dill, ground flaxseeds, and dried barberries, all ready to spontaneously add extra texture, flavor, and nutrition to meals.

It takes time to build up a truly plant-terrific kitchen, and I recommend going at whatever pace you feel comfortable to transition to a fully evidence-based diet. The people who try to adopt a whole-food, plant-based diet cold turkey are often, I'm afraid, the ones who may not keep it up. People who learn to eat well over time, food by food and meal by meal, may do best. They experiment with new foods, deliberately adding more vegetables to their diet to crowd out some of the less healthy choices and when they can, introducing a new, healthful recipe to their cooking repertoire. Then they find another such recipe, and another, until all of their meals are centered around Green Light foods.

The most important thing to keep in mind is long-term sustainability. It's not what you ate for the first few decades of your life, or even what you eat tomorrow or next week, that matters. It's all about what you eat for the next few decades. So please proceed at whatever pace works best for you. Remember: don't stress if you fall off the wagon from time to time. If you do eat poorly one day, simply try to eat better the next.

Besides these basics, it's also important to find foods you love. And the best way to do that may be to expand your horizons. There are all kinds of exotic beans and greens, so why not select some you aren't as familiar with? How about adzuki beans or gigantes? What about sorrel or kai-lan (Chinese broccoli)? If you're lucky enough to have a large Asian market near you, that's where you can find more unusual produce, such as jackfruit, which looks like a huge, spiky melon with a shredded meatlike texture that can help extend your meatless Monday health streak into taco Tuesday. Although eating healthfully might sound limiting at first, many people tell me that they end up eating a more diverse diet than they ever have before.

Venture into the ethnic sections of your local markets, which span Mexican, Chinese, Indian, Thai, Ethiopian, and beyond. The goal is to find sauces or seasonings that can jazz up the most humble of beans or greens. Most prepared sauces are Yellow or Red Light foods, with added salt, sugar, and fat, but if a not-so-good-for-you sauce dramatically increases your intake of whole plant foods, it may be worth it to use it until you can Google your way to find a Green Light alternative.

Some spice mixes may start out in the Green, such as Italian, jerk, taco, berbere, garam masala, and za'atar. Be sure to have some on hand so when you're in the midst of cooking, you can just toss some in the pot without having to worry about the proper ratio of basil-to-oregano (or whatever). That's already been taken care of for you.

To help you stock your pantry, the following list is a guide to the foods you may want to have, particularly if you are going to be cooking up the recipes in this book.

PANTRY

artichoke hearts (jarred or frozen)

BEANS: (dried and canned) black beans, chickpeas, kidney beans, navy beans, black-eyed peas, pinto beans, lentils, split peas, and cannellini beans

chickpea flour

chipotle chilies in adobo

cocoa powder (unsweetened)

curry powder

date sugar

dried chilies

DRIED FRUITS: dates, raisins, apricots, goji berries, figs

dulse seaweed flakes

GRAINS: red, brown, or black rice, red or black quinoa, old-fashioned rolled oats

miso paste (white)

mustard (salt-free stone-ground)

nut butters and tahini

nutritional yeast

NUTS AND SEEDS: cashews, almonds, pecans, peanuts, walnuts, flaxseeds, sesame seeds, hulled hemp seeds (hemp hearts)

PASTA AND NOODLES: 100% whole-grain or bean-based spaghetti, linguine, fusilli, lasagna, soba

roasted red peppers, jarred

spices and dried herbs

TOMATO PRODUCTS: salt-free jarred, BPA-free canned, or Tetra Pak tomato products (diced, whole, purée, paste, marinara sauce)

TORTILLAS: 100% whole-grain and corn

vanilla beans

vinegars (balsamic, rice, tarragon)

FRESH

FRUITS AND ROOT VEGETABLES: onions, garlic, carrots, sweet potatoes, and celery, as well as lemons, limes, bananas, gingerroot, and seasonal fruits

LEAFY GREENS: kale, baby spinach, arugula, and fresh herbs, as well as crucifers including cauliflower and purple cabbage

SALAD INGREDIENTS: lettuce, cucumber, tomato, bell pepper, and avocado, and other vegetables, such as asparagus, green beans, broccoli, mushrooms, squash, and corn

tempeh

FROZEN

VEGETABLES: greens, corn kernels, green peas, edamame

FRUIT: blueberries, cherries, strawberries, peaches, mangoes

cooked and portioned rice (black, red, or brown), beans, and Vegetable Broth (page 6)

ALSO, KEEP ON HAND THE FOLLOWING:

Almond Milk (page 2)

Date Syrup (page 3)

Savory Spice Blend (page 4)

Nutty Parm (page 4)

Umami Sauce (page 5)

Vegetable Broth (page 6)

Healthy Hot Sauce (page 8)

REFERENCES

1. D. Ornish, S. E. Brown, L. W. Scherwitz, et al., "Can Lifestyle Changes Reverse Coronary Heart Disease? The Lifestyle Heart Trial," *Lancet* 336, no. 8707 (1990): 129–33.

2. J. W. Anderson and K. Ward, "High-Carbohydrate, High-Fiber Diets for Insulin-Treated Men with Diabetes Mellitus," *Am J Clin Nutr* 32, no. 11 (1979): 2312–21.

3. Kaiser Permanente, "The Plant-Based Diet: A Healthier Way to Eat," https://share.kaiserpermanente.org/wp-content/uploads/2015/10/The-Plant-Based-Diet-booklet.pdf. 2013, accessed April 10, 2015.

4. T. Monte and I. Pritikin, *Pritikin: The Man Who Healed America's Heart* (Emmaus, PA: Rodale Press; 1988).

5. D. Mozaffarian, E. J. Benjamin, A. S. Go, et al., "Heart Disease and Stroke Statistics—2015 Update: A Report from the American Heart Association," *Circulation* 131, no. 4 (2015): e29–322.

6. T. C. Campbell, B. Parpia, and J. Chen, "Diet, Lifestyle, and the Etiology of Coronary Artery Disease: The Cornell China Study," *Am J Cardiol* 82, no. 10B (1998): 18T–21T.

7. W. A. Thomas, J. N. Davies, R. M. O'Neal, and A. A. Dimakulangan, "Incidence of Myocardial Infarction Correlated with Venous and Pulmonary Thrombosis and Embolism. A Geographic Study Based on Autopsies in Uganda, East Africa and St. Louis, U.S.A.," *Am J Cardiol* 5 (1960): 41–47.

8. R. D. Voller and W. B. Strong, "Pediatric Aspects of Atherosclerosis," *Am Heart J* 101, no. 6 (1981): 815–36.

9. C. Napoli, F. P. D'Armiento, FP. Mancini, et al., "Fatty Streak Formation Occurs in Human Fetal Aortas and Is Greatly Enhanced by Maternal Hypercholesterolemia. Intimal Accumulation of Low Density Lipoprotein and Its Oxidation Precede Monocyte Recruitment into Early Atherosclerotic Lesions," *J Clin Invest* 100, no. 11 (1997): 2680–90.

10. W. F. Enos, R. H. Holmes, and J. Beyer, "Coronary Disease Among United States Soldiers Killed in Action in Korea: Preliminary Report," *J Am Med Assoc* 152, no. 12 (1953): 1090–93.

11. R. D. Voller and W. B. Strong, "Pediatric Aspects of Atherosclerosis," *Am Heart J* 101, no. 6 (1981): 815–36.

12. D. Ornish, L. W. Scherwitz, J. H. Billings, et al., "Intensive Lifestyle Changes for Reversal of Coronary Heart Disease," *JAMA* 280, no. 23 (1998): 2001–7.

13. C. B. Esselstyn Jr, G. Gendy, J. Doyle, M. Golubic, and M. F. Roizen, "A Way to Reverse CAD?" *J Fam Pract* 63, no. 7 (2014): 356–64b.

14. American Cancer Society, "Cancer Facts and Figures 2015" (Atlanta: American Cancer Society, 2015); National Heart, Lung, and Blood Institute, NIH, *NHLBI Fact Book, Fiscal Year 2012*, http://www.nhlbi.nih.gov/files/docs/factbook/FactBook2012.pdf, February 2013, accessed March 31, 2015.

15. P. Riso, D. Martini, P. Møller, et al., "DNA Damage and Repair Activity After Broccoli Intake in Young Healthy Smokers," *Mutagenesis* 25, no. 6 (November 2010): 595–602.

16. I. C. Walda, C. Tabak, H. A. Smit, et al., "Diet and 20-Year Chronic Obstructive Pulmonary Disease Mortality in Middle-Aged Men from Three European Countries," *Eur J Clin Nutr* 56, no. 7 (2002): 638–43.

17. J. L. Protudjer, G. P. Sevenhuysen, C. D. Ramsey, A. L. Kozyrskyj, and A. B. Becker, "Low Vegetable Intake Is Associated with Allergic Asthma and Moderate-to-Severe Airway Hyperresponsiveness," *Pediatr Pulmonol* 47, no. 12 (2012): 1159–69.

18. L. G. Wood, M. L. Garg, J. M. Smart, H. A. Scott, D. Barker, and P. G. Gibson, "Manipulating Antioxidant Intake in Asthma: A Randomized Controlled Trial," *Am J Clin Nutr* 96, no. 3 (2012): 534–43.

19. D. Mozaffarian, E. J. Benjamin, A. S. Go, et al., "Heart Disease and Stroke Statistics—2015 Update: A Report from the American Heart Association," *Circulation* 131, no. 4 (2015): e29–322; Centers for Disease Control and Prevention, Deaths: Final Data for 2013 Table 10, "Number of deaths from 113 selected causes," *National Vital Statistics Report 2016* 64, no. 2.

20. D. E. Threapleton, D. C. Greenwood, C. E. Evans, et al., "Dietary Fiber Intake and Risk of First Stroke: A Systematic Review and Meta-analysis," *Stroke* 44, no. 5 (2013): 1360–68.

21. L. D'Elia, G. Barba, F. P. Cappuccio, and P. Strazzullo, "Potassium Intake, Stroke, and Cardiovascular Disease: A Meta-analysis of Prospective Studies," *J Am Coll Cardiol* 57, no. 10 (2011): 1210–19.

22. J. C. de la Torre, "Alzheimer's Disease Is Incurable but Preventable," *J Alzheimers Dis* 20, no. 3 (2010): 861–70.

23 A. E. Roher, S. L. Tyas, C. L. Maarouf, et al., "Intracranial Atherosclerosis as a Contributing Factor to Alzheimer's Disease Dementia," *Alzheimers Dement* 7, no. 4 (2011): 436–44; M. Yarchoan, S. X. Xie, M. A. Kling, et al., "Cerebrovascular Atherosclerosis Correlates with Alzheimer Pathology in Neurodegenerative Dementias," *Brain* 135, part 2 (2012): 3749–56; L. S. Honig, W. Kukull, and R. Mayeux, "Atherosclerosis and AD: Analysis of Data from the US National Alzheimer's Coordinating Center," *Neurology* 64, no. 3 (2005): 494–500.

24 L. White, H. Petrovitch, G. W. Ross, et al., Prevalence of Dementia in Older Japanese-American Men in Hawaii: The Honolulu-Asia Aging Study," *JAMA* 276, no. 12 (1996): 955–60.

25 H. C. Hendrie, A. Ogunniyi, K. S. Hall, et al., "Incidence of Dementia and Alzheimer Disease in 2 Communities: Yoruba Residing in Ibadan, Nigeria, and African Americans Residing in Indianapolis, Indiana," *JAMA* 285, no. 6 (2001): 739–47.

26 V. Chandra, M. Ganguli, R. Pandav, et al., "Prevalence of Alzheimer's Disease and Other Dementias in Rural India: The Indo-US Study," *Neurology* 51, no. 4 (1998): 1000–1008.

27 P. S. Shetty, "Nutrition Transition in India," *Public Health Nutr* 5, no. 1A (2002): 175–82.

28 American Cancer Society, "Cancer Facts and Figures 2015," Atlanta: American Cancer Society, 2015.

29 T. T. Macdonald and G. Monteleone, "Immunity, Inflammation, and Allergy in the Gut," *Science* 307. no. 5717 (2005): 1920–25.

30 S. Bengmark, M. D. Mesa, and A. Gill, "Plant-Derived Health—The Effects of Turmeric and Curcuminoids," *Nutr Hosp* 24, no. 3 (2009): 273–81.

31 A. Hutchins-Wolfbrandt and A. M. Mistry, "Dietary Turmeric Potentially Reduces the Risk of Cancer," *Asian Pac J Cancer Prev* 12, no. 12 (2011): 3169–73.

32 International Institute for Population Sciences (IIPS) and Macro International. *National Family Health Survey (NFHS-3), 2005-06: India: Volume. 1.* Mumbai: IIPS, 2007. http://dhsprogram.com/pubs/pdf/FRIND3/FRIND3-Vol1andVol2.pdf

33 American Cancer Society, "Cancer Facts and Figures 2014," Atlanta: American Cancer Society, 2014.

34 A. C. Thiébaut, L. Jiao, D. T. Silverman, et al., "Dietary Fatty Acids and Pancreatic Cancer in the NIH-AARP Diet and Health Study," *J Natl Cancer Inst* 101, no. 14 (2009): 1001–11.

35 S. Rohrmann, J. Linseisen, U. Nöthlings, et al., "Meat and Fish Consumption and Risk of Pancreatic Cancer: Results from the European Prospective Investigation into Cancer and Nutrition," *Int J Cancer* 132, no. 3 (2013): 617–24.

36 Centers for Disease Control and Prevention, "Deaths: Final Data for 2013 Table 10."

37 A. Gibson, J. Edgar, C. Neville, et al., "Effect of Fruit and Vegetable Consumption on Immune Function in Older People: A Randomized Controlled Trial," *Am J Clin Nutr* 96, no. 6 (2012): 1429–36.

38 M. Veldhoen, "Direct Interactions Between Intestinal Immune Cells and the Diet," *Cell Cycle* 11, no. 3 (February 1, 2012): 426–27.

39 L. S. McAnulty, D. C. Nieman, C. L. Dumke, et al., "Effect of Blueberry Ingestion on Natural Killer Cell Counts, Oxidative Stress, and Inflammation Prior to and after 2.5 H of Running," *Appl Physiol Nutr Metab* 36, no. 6 (2011): 976–84.

40 Centers for Disease Control and Prevention, "Number (in Millions) of Civilian, Noninstitutionalized Persons with Diagnosed Diabetes, United States, 1980–2011," http://www.cdc.gov/diabetes/statistics/prev/national/figpersons.htm, March 28, 2013, accessed May 3, 2015.

41 Centers for Disease Control and Prevention, "Deaths: Final Data for 2013 Table 10."

42 M. Roden, T. B. Price, G. Perseghin, et al., "Mechanism of Free Fatty Acid–Induced Insulin Resistance in Humans," *J Clin Invest* 97, no. 12 (1996): 2859–65.

43 E. Ginter and V. Simko, "Type 2 Diabetes Mellitus, Pandemic in 21st Century," *Adv Exp Med Biol* 771 (2012): 42–50.

44 S. Tonstad, T. Butler, R. Yan, and G. E. Fraser, "Type of Vegetarian Diet, Body Weight, and Prevalence of Type 2 Diabetes," *Diabetes Care* 32, no. 5 (2009): 791–96.

45 R. C. Mollard, B. L. Luhovyy, S. Panahi, M. Nunez, A. Hanley, and G. H. Anderson, "Regular Consumption of Pulses for 8 Weeks Reduces Metabolic Syndrome Risk Factors in Overweight and Obese Adults," *Br J Nutr* 108, suppl. 1 (2012): S111–22.

46 S. Tonstad, K. Stewart, K. Oda, M. Batech, R. P. Herring, and G. E. Fraser, "Vegetarian Diets and Incidence of Diabetes in the Adventist Health Study-2," *Nutr Metab Cardiovasc Dis* 23, no. 4 (2013): 292–99.

47 J. W. Anderson and K. Ward, "High-Carbohydrate, High-Fiber Diets for Insulin-Treated Men with Diabetes Mellitus," *Am J Clin Nutr* 32, no. 11 (1979): 2312–21.

48 S. Bromfield and P. Muntner, "High Blood Pressure: The Leading Global Burden of Disease Risk Factor and the Need for Worldwide Prevention Programs," *Curr Hypertens Rep* 15, no. 3 (2013): 134–36.

49 S. S. Lim, T. Vos, A. D. Flaxman, et al., "A Comparative Risk Assessment of Burden of Disease and Injury Attributable to 67 Risk Factors and Risk Factor Clusters in 21 Regions, 1990–2010: A Systematic Analysis for the Global Burden of Disease Study 2010," *Lancet* 380, no. 9859 (2012): 2224–60.

50 D. Mozaffarian, E. J. Benjamin, A. S. Go, et al., "Heart Disease and Stroke Statistics—2015 Update: A Report from the American Heart Association," *Circulation* 131, no. 4 (2015): e29–322.

51 T. Nwankwo, S. S. Yoon, V. Burt, and Q. Gu, "Hypertension among Adults in the United States: National Health and Nutrition Examination Survey, 2011–2012," *NCHS Data Brief* no. 133 (2013): 1–8.

52 C. P. Donnison, "Blood Pressure in the African Native," *Lancet* 213, no. 5497 (1929): 6–7.

53 M. R. Law, J. K. Morris, and N. J. Wald, "Use of Blood Pressure Lowering Drugs in the Prevention of Cardiovascular Disease: Meta-analysis of 147 Randomised Trials in the Context of Expectations from Prospective Epidemiological Studies," *BMJ* 338 (2009): b1665.

54 P. Tighe, G. Duthie, N. Vaughan, et al., "Effect of Increased Consumption of Whole-Grain Foods on Blood Pressure and Other Cardiovascular Risk Markers in Healthy Middle-Aged Persons: A Randomized Controlled Trial," *Am J Clin Nutr* 92, no. 4 (2010): 733–40.

55 D. L. McKay, C. Y. Chen, E. Saltzman, and J. B. Blumberg, "*Hibiscus sabdariffa* L. tea (Tisane) Lowers Blood Pressure in Prehypertensive and Mildly Hypertensive Adults," *J Nutr* 140. no. 2 (2010): 298–303.

56 D. Rodriguez-Leyva, W. Weighell, A. L. Edel, et al., "Potent Antihypertensive Action of Dietary Flaxseed in Hypertensive Patients," *Hypertension* 62, no. 6 (2013): 1081–89.

57 Centers for Disease Control and Prevention, "Deaths: Final Data for 2013 Table 10."

58 E. M. McCarthy and M. E. Rinella, "The Role of Diet and Nutrient Composition in Nonalcoholic Fatty Liver Disease," *J Acad Nutr Diet* 112, no. 3 (2012): 401–9.

59 J. F. Silverman, W. J. Pories, and J. F. Caro, "Liver Pathology in Diabetes Mellitus and Morbid Obesity: Clinical, Pathological and Biochemical Considerations," *Pathol Annu* 24 (1989): 275–302.

60 S. Singh, A. M. Allen, Z. Wang, L. J. Prokop, M. H. Murad, and R. Loomba, "Fibrosis Progression in Nonalcoholic Fatty Liver vs Nonalcoholic Steatohepatitis: A Systematic Review and Meta-analysis of Paired-Biopsy Studies," *Clin Gastroenterol Hepatol* S1542–3565, no. 14 (2014), 00602–8.

61 S. Zelber-Sagi, D. Nitzan-Kaluski, R. Goldsmith, et al., "Long Term Nutritional Intake and the Risk for Non-alcoholic Fatty Liver Disease (NAFLD): A Population Based Study," *J Hepatol* 47, no. 5 (November 2007): 711–17.

62 Ibid.

63 H. C. Chang, C. N. Huang, D. M. Yeh, S. J. Wang, C. H. Peng, and C. J. Wang, "Oat Prevents Obesity and Abdominal Fat Distribution, and Improves Liver Function in Humans," *Plant Foods Hum Nutr* 68, no. 1 (2013): 18–23.

64 American Cancer Society, "Cancer Facts and Figures 2015."

65 T. J. Key, P. N. Appleby, E. A. Spencer, et al., "Cancer Incidence in British Vegetarians," *Br J Cancer* 101, no. 1 (2009): 192–97.

66 C. A. Thompson, T. M. Habermann, A. H. Wang, et al., "Antioxidant Intake from Fruits, Vegetables and Other Sources and Risk of Non-Hodgkin's Lymphoma: The Iowa Women's Health Study," *Int J Cancer* 136, no. 4 (2010): 992–1003.

67 S. G. Holtan, H. M. O'Connor, Z. S. Fredericksen, et al., "Food-Frequency Questionnaire-Based Estimates of Total Antioxidant Capacity and Risk of Non-Hodgkin Lymphoma," *Int J Cancer* 131, no. 5 (2012;): 1158–68.

68 Centers for Disease Control and Prevention. "Deaths: Final Data for 2013 Table 10."

69 J. Coresh, E. Selvin, L. A. Stevens, et al., "Prevalence of Chronic Kidney Disease in the United States," *JAMA* 298, no. 17 (2007): 2038–47.

70 T. P. Ryan, J. A. Sloand, P. C. Winters, J. P. Corsetti, and S. G. Fisher, "Chronic Kidney Disease Prevalence and Rate of Diagnosis," *Am J Med* 120, no. 11 (2007): 981–86.

71 J. Lin, F. B. Hu, And G. C. Curhan, "Associations of Diet with Albuminuria and Kidney Function Decline," *Clin J Am Soc Nephrol* 5, no. 5 (2010): 836–43.

72 P. Fioretto, R. Trevisan, A. Valerio, et al., "Impaired Renal Response to a Meat Meal in Insulin-Dependent Diabetes: Role of Glucagon and Prostaglandins," *Am J Physiol* 258, no. 3, part 2 (1990): F675–F83.

73 A. H. Simon, P. R. Lima, M. Almerinda V. F. Alves, P. V. Bottini, and J. B. Lopes de Faria, "Renal Haemodynamic Responses to a Chicken or Beef Meal in Normal Individuals," *Nephrol Dial Transplant* 13, no. 9 (1998): 2261–64.

74 P. Kontessis, S. Jones, R. Dodds, et al., "Renal, Metabolic and Hormonal Responses to Ingestion of Animal and Vegetable Proteins," *Kidney Int* 38, no. 1 (July 1990): 136–44.

75 Z. M. Liu, S. C. Ho, Y. M. Chen, N. Tang, and J. Woo, "Effect of Whole Soy and Purified Isoflavone Daidzein on Renal Function—A 6-Month Randomized Controlled Trial in Equol-Producing Postmenopausal Women with Prehypertension," *Clin Biochem* 47, nos. 13–14 (2014): 1250–56.

76 American Cancer Society, "Breast Cancer Facts and Figures 2013–2014," http://www.cancer.org/acs/groups/content/@research/documents/document/acspc-042725.pdf, published 2013, accessed March 10, 2015.

77 S. E. Steck, M. M. Gaudet, S. M. Eng, et al., "Cooked Meat and Risk of Breast Cancer—Lifetime versus Recent Dietary Intake," *Epidemiology* 18, no. 3 (2007): 373–82.

78 C. M. Kitahara, A. Berrington de Gonzhara, N. D. Freedman, et al., "Total Cholesterol and Cancer Risk in a Large Prospective Study in Korea," *J Clin Oncol* 29, no. 12 (2011): 1592–98.

79 D. A. Boggs, J. R. Palmer, L. A. Wise, et al., "Fruit and Vegetable Intake in Relation to Risk of Breast Cancer in the Black Women's Health Study," *Am J Epidemiol* 172, no. 11 (2010): 1268–79.

80 Q. Li, T. R. Holford, Y. Zhang, et al., "Dietary Fiber Intake and Risk of Breast Cancer by Menopausal and Estrogen Receptor Status," *Eur J Nutr* 52, no. 1 (2013): 217–23.

81 Centers for Disease Control and Prevention, "Deaths: Final Data for 2013, table 18," http://www.cdc.gov/nchs/data/nvsr/nvsr64/nvsr64_02.pdf, accessed March 20, 2015.

82 N. Sartorius, "The Economic and Social Burden of Depression," *J Clin Psychiatry*, 62, suppl. 15 (2001): 8–11.

83 A. C. Tsai, T.-L. Chang, and S.-H. Chi, "Frequent Consumption of Vegetables Predicts Lower Risk of Depression in Older Taiwanese—Results of a Prospective Population-Based Study," *Public Health Nutr* 15, no. 6 (2012): 1087–92.

84 F. Gomez-Pinilla and T. T. J. Nguyen, "Natural Mood Foods: The Actions of Polyphenols against Psychiatric and Cognitive Disorders," *Nutr Neurosci* 15, no. 3 (2012): 127–33.

85 A. A. Noorbala, S. Akhondzadeh, N. Tahmacebi-Pour, and A. H. Jamshidi, "Hydro-alcoholic Extract of Crocus sativus L. versus Fluoxetine in the Treatment of Mild to Moderate Depression: A Double-Blind, Randomized Pilot Trial," *J Ethnopharmacol* 97, no. 2 (2005): 281–84.

86 J. L. Jahn, E. L. Giovannucci, and M. J. Stampfer, "The High Prevalence of Undiagnosed Prostate Cancer at Autopsy: Implications for Epidemiology and Treatment of Prostate Cancer in the Prostate-Specific Antigen-Era," *Int J Cancer* 137, no. 12 (2015): 2795-2802.

87 Centers for Disease Control and Prevention, "Prostate Cancer Statistics," http://www.cdc.gov/cancer/prostate/statistics/index.htm, updated September 2, 2014, accessed March 11, 2015.

88 D. Ganmaa, X. M. Li, L. Q. Qin, P. Y. Wang, M. Takeda, and A. Sato," "The Experience of Japan as a Clue to the Etiology of Testicular and Prostatic Cancers," *Med Hypotheses* 60, no. 5 (2003): 724–30.

89 D. Aune, D. A. Navarro Rosenblatt, D. S. Chan, et al., "Dairy Products, Calcium, and Prostate Cancer Risk: A Systematic Review and Meta-analysis of Cohort Studies," *Am J Clin Nutr* 101, no. 1 (2015): 87–117.

90 D. Ornish, G. Weidner, W. R. Fair, et al., "Intensive Lifestyle Changes May Affect the Progression of Prostate Cancer," *J Urol* 174, no. 3 (2005): 1065–69.

91 Centers for Disease Control and Prevention, "Deaths: Final Data for 2013, table 10."

92 R. Vogt, D. Bennett, D. Cassady, J. Frost, B. Ritz, and I. Hertz-Picciotto, "Cancer and Non-cancer Health Effects from Food Contaminant Exposures for Children and Adults in California: A Risk Assessment," *Environ Health* 11 (2012): 83.

93 European Food Safety Authority, "Results of the Monitoring of Non Dioxin-like PCBs in Food and Feed," *EFSA Journal* 8, no. 7 (2010): 1701.

94 H. Arguin, M. Arguin, G. A. Bray, et al., "Impact of Adopting a Vegan Diet or an Olestra Supplementation on Plasma Organochlorine Concentrations: Results from Two Pilot Studies," *Br J Nutr* 103, no. 10 (2010): 1433–41.

95 J. Lazarou, B. H. Pomeranz, and P. N. Corey, "Incidence of Adverse Drug Reactions in Hospitalized Patients: A Meta-analysis of Prospective Studies," *JAMA* 279, no. 15 (1998): 1200–1205; B. Starfield, "Is US Health Really the Best in the World?," *JAMA* 284, no. 4 (2000): 483–85; R. M. Klevens, J. R. Edwards, C. L. Richards, et al., "Estimating Health Care–Associated Infections and Deaths in U.S. Hospitals, 2002," *Public Health Rep* 122, no. 2 (2007): 160–66; Institute of Medicine, "To Err Is Human: Building a Safer Health System," http://www.iom.edu/~/media/Files/Report%20Files/1999/To-Err-is-Human/To%20Err%20is%20Human%201999%20%20report%20brief.pdf, November 1999, accessed March 12, 2015.

96 Klevens, Edwards, Richards, et al., "Estimating Health Care–Associated Infections and Deaths in U.S. Hospitals, 2002."

97 Lazarou, Pomeranz, and Corey, "Incidence of Adverse Drug Reactions in Hospitalized Patients."

98 Institute of Medicine, "To Err Is Human."

99 E. Picano, "Informed Consent and Communication of Risk from Radiological and Nuclear Medicine Examinations: How to Escape from a Communication Inferno," *BMJ* 329, no. 7470 (2004): 849–51.

100 C. W. Schmidt, "CT Scans: Balancing Health Risks and Medical Benefits," *Environ Health Perspect* 120, no. 3 (2012): A118–21.

101 P. N. Trewby, A. V. Reddy, C. S. Trewby, V. J. Ashton, G. Brennan, and J. Inglis, "Are Preventive Drugs Preventive Enough? A Study of Patients' Expectation of Benefit from Preventive Drugs," *Clin Med* 2, no. 6 (2002): 527–33.

102 Y. F. Chu, J. Sun, X. Wu, and R. H. Liu, "Antioxidant and Antiproliferative Activities of Common Vegetables," *J Agric Food Chem* 50, no. 23 (2002): 6910–16.

103 W. Rock, M. Rosenblat, H. Borochov-Neori, N. Volkova, S. Judeinstein, M. Elias, and M. Aviram, Effects of Date (Phoenix dactylifera L., Medjool or Hallawi Variety) Consumption by Healthy Subjects on Serum Glucose and Lipid Levels and on Serum Oxidative Status: A Pilot Study," *J Agric Food Chem* 57, no. 17 (September 9, 2009): 8010–17.

104 D. Rodriguez-Leyva, W. Weighell, A. L. Edel, et al., "Potent Antihypertensive Action of Dietary Flaxseed in Hypertensive Patients," *Hypertension* 62, no. 6 (2013): 1081–89.

105 V. A. Cornelissen, R. Buys, and N. A. Smart, "Endurance Exercise Beneficially Affects Ambulatory Blood Pressure: A Systematic Review and Meta-analysis," *J Hypertens* 31, no. 4 (2013): 639–48.

106 C. J. Fabian, B. F. Kimler, C. M. Zalles, et al., "Reduction in Ki-67 in Benign Breast Tissue of High-Risk Women with the Lignan Secoisolariciresinol Diglycoside," *Cancer Prev Res* (Phila) 3, no. 10 (2010): 1342–50.

107 S. Y. Kim, S. Yoon, S. M. Kwon, K. S. Park, and Y. C. Lee-kim, "Kale Juice Improves Coronary Artery Disease Risk Factors in Hypercholesterolemic Men," *Biomed Environ Sci* 21, no. 2 (2008): 91–97.

108 R. H. Dressendorfer, C. E. Wade, C. Hornick, and G. C. Timmis, "High-Density Lipoprotein-Cholesterol in Marathon Runners during a 20-Day Road Race," *JAMA* 247, no. 12 (1982): 1715–17.

109 G. K. Hovingh, D. J. Rader, and R. A. Hegele, "HDL Re-examined," *Curr Opin Lipidol* 26, no. 2 (2015): 127–32.

110 D. B. Haytowitz and S. A. Bhagwat, "USDA Database for the Oxygen Radical Capacity (ORAC) of Selected Foods, Release 2," Washington, DC: United States Department of Agriculture, 2010.

111 U.S. Department of Agriculture, "Oxygen Radical Absorbance Capacity (ORAC) of Selected Foods—2007," http://www.orac-info-portal.de/download/ORAC_R2.pdf, November 2007, accessed April 10, 2015.

112 R. C. Mollard, B. L. Luhovyy, S. Panahi, M. Nunez, A. Hanley, and G. H. Anderson, "Regular Consumption of Pulses for 8 Weeks Reduces Metabolic Syndrome Risk Factors in Overweight and Obese Adults," *Br J Nutr* 108, suppl. 1 (2012): S111–22.

113 H. C. Hung, K. J. Joshipura, R. Jiang, et al., "Fruit and Vegetable Intake and Risk of Major Chronic Disease," *J Natl Cancer Inst* 96, no. 21 (2004): 1577–84.

114 K. J. Joshipura, F. B. Hu, J. E. Manson, et al., "The Effect of Fruit and Vegetable Intake on Risk for Coronary Heart Disease," *Ann Intern Med* 134, no. 12 (2001): 1106–14.

115 K. J. Joshipura, A. Ascherio, J. E. Manson, et al., "Fruit and Vegetable Intake in Relation to Risk of Ischemic Stroke," *JAMA* 282, no. 13 (1999): 1233–39.

116 Y. F. Chu, J. Sun, X. Wu, and R. H. Liu, "Antioxidant and Antiproliferative Activities of Common Vegetables," *J Agric Food Chem* 50, no. 23 (2002): 6910–16.

117 M. N. Chen, C. C. Lin, and C. F. Liu, "Efficacy of Phytoestrogens for Menopausal Symptoms: A Meta-analysis and Systematic Review," *Climacteric* 18, no. 2 (2015): 260–69.

118 C. Nagata, T. Mizoue, K. Tanaka, et al., "Soy Intake and Breast Cancer Risk: An Evaluation Based on a Systematic Review of Epidemiologic Evidence among the Japanese Population," *Jpn J Clin Oncol* 44, no. 3 (2014): 282–95.

119 F. Chi, R. Wu, Y. C. Zeng, R. Xing, Y. Liu, and Z. G. Xu, "Post-diagnosis Soy Food Intake and Breast Cancer Survival: A Meta-analysis of Cohort Studies," *Asian Pac J Cancer Prev* 14, no. 4 (2013): 2407–12.

120 E. L. Richman, P. R. Carroll, and J. M. Chan, "Vegetable and Fruit Intake after Diagnosis and Risk of Prostate Cancer Progression," *Int J Cancer* 131, no. 1 (2012): 201–10.

121 S. S. Nielsen, G. M. Franklin, W. T. Longstreth, P. D. Swanson, and H. Checkoway, "Nicotine from Edible Solanaceae and Risk of Parkinson Disease," *Ann Neurol* 74, no. 3 (2013): 472–77.

122 Y. F. Chu, J. Sun, X. Wu, and R. H. Liu, "Antioxidant and Antiproliferative Activities of Common Vegetables," *J Agric Food Chem* 50, no. 23 (2002): 6910–16.

123 S. C. Jeong, S. R. Koyyalamudi, and G. Pang, "Dietary Intake of Agaricusbisporus White Button Mushroom Accelerates Salivary Immunoglobulin A Secretion in Healthy Volunteers," *Nutrition* 28, no. 5 (2012): 527–31.

124 M. Jesenak, M. Hrubisko, J. Majtan, Z. Rennerova, and P. Banovcin, "Anti-allergic Effect of Pleuran (β-glucan from Pleurotus ostreatus) in Children with Recurrent Respiratory Tract Infections," *Phyto-ther Res* 28, no. 3 (2014): 471–74.

125 M. Maghbooli, F. Golipour, A. Moghimi Esfandabadi, and M. Yousefi, "Comparison between the Efficacy of Ginger and Sumatriptan in the Ablative Treatment of the Common Migraine," *Phytother Res* 28, no. 3 (2014): 412–15.

126 F. Kashefi, M. Khajehei, M. Tabatabaeichehr, M. Alavinia, and J. Asili, "Comparison of the Effect of Ginger and Zinc Sulfate on Primary Dysmenorrhea: A Placebo-Controlled Randomized Trial," *Pain Manag Nurs* 15, no. 4 (2014): 826–33.

127 World Cancer Research Fund/American Institute for Cancer Research, "Food, Nutrition, Physical Activity, and the Prevention of Cancer: A Global Perspective," Washington, DC: AICR, 2007.

128 G. E. Fraser and D. J. Shavlik, "Ten Years of Life: Is It a Matter of Choice?" *Arch Intern Med* 181, no. 13 (2001): 1645–52.

129 N. Annema, J. S. Heyworth, S. A. Mcnaughton, B. Iacopetta, and L. Fritschi, "Fruit and Vegetable Consumption and the Risk of Proximal Colon, Distal Colon, and Rectal Cancers in a Case-Control Study in Western Australia," *J Am Diet Assoc* 111, no. 10 (2011): 1479–90.

130 Y. F. Chu, J. Sun, X. Wu, and R. H. Liu, "Antioxidant and Antiproliferative Activities of Common Vegetables," *J Agric Food Chem* 50, no. 23 (2002): 6910–16.

131 M. Murphy, K. Eliot, R. M. Heuertz, and E. Weiss, "Whole Beetroot Consumption Acutely Improves Running Performance," *J Acad Nutr Diet* 111, no. 4 (2012): 548–52.

132 V. Kapil, R. S. Khambata, A. Robertson, M. J. Caulfield, and A. Ahluwalia, "Dietary Nitrate Provides Sustained Blood Pressure Lowering in Hypertensive Patients: A Randomized, Phase 2, Double-Blind, Placebo-Controlled Study," *Hypertension* 65, no. 2 (2015): 320–27.

133 M. Cruz-Correa, D. A. Shoskes, P. Sanchez, et al., "Combination Treatment with Curcumin and Quercetin of Adenomas in Familial Adenomatous Polyposis," *Clin Gastroenterol Hepatol* 4, no. 8 (2006): 1035–38.

134 C. Galeone, C. Pelucchi, R. Talamini, et al., "Onion and Garlic Intake and the Odds of Benign Prostatic Hyperplasia," *Urology* 70, no. 4 (2007): 672–76.

135 S. Gallus, R. Talamini, A. Giacosa, et al., "Does an Apple a Day Keep the Oncologist Away?" *Ann Oncol* 16, no. 11 (2005): 1841–44.

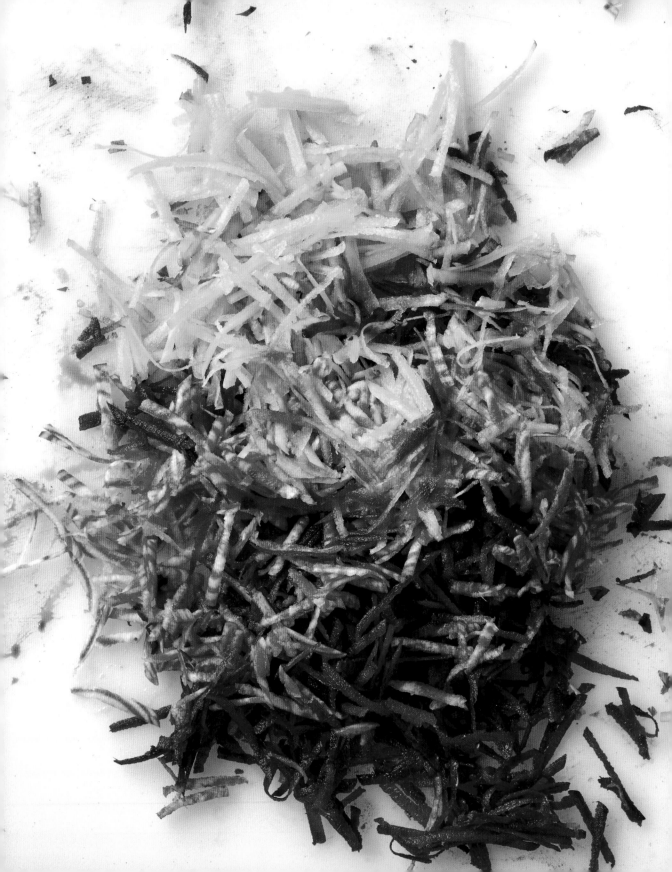

INDEX

Page numbers in italic indicate photographs.

A

Advanced glycation end products (AGEs), 108
Africa, xiv, 9, 118, 124
African American women, xviii
AGEs. *See* Advanced glycation end products
Almonds
    almond butter, 2
    Almond Butter Sauce, 146
    Almond Milk, xi, 2, 7, 12, 16, 22, 111, 121, 130,
        180, 200, 209
    Almond-Chocolate Truffles, *186*, 187
Alzheimer's disease, xiii–xiv
Antidepressants, xviii
Antioxidants, xvii, 8, 30, 56, 59, 76, 106, 108, 227
Appetizers, 28–29
    Artichoke-Spinach Dip, 30, *31*
    Black-Eyed Peas & Roasted Red Pepper Dip, 36, *37*
    Cheesy Kale Crisps, 42, *43*
    Edamame Guacamole, 38, *39*
    Lemony Hummus, *32*, 33
    Pumpkin Seed Dip, 35
    Smoky Roasted Chickpeas, 44, *45*
    Summer Salsa, *40*, 41
    Three-Seed Crackers, 34
Apples
    Baked Apple Crumbles, 190, *191*
    benefits from, 190
Arrabiata, 108, *109*
Arthritis, 70
Artichoke-Spinach Dip, 30, *31*
Arugula Pesto Pasta with Roasted Vegetables, *160*, 161

Asparagus, 164, *165*
Asthma, xiii
Atherosclerotic plaque buildup, xiv
Avocado
    Avocado Goddess Dressing, 72, *73*
    Avocado-Cashew Alfredo, *104*, 105
    Edamame Guacamole, 38, *39*
    Mango-Avocado-Kale Salad with Ginger Sesame
        Orange Dressing, 80, *81*

B

B vitamins, x
Bacteria, xv
Bahri dates, 8
Baked Apple Crumbles, 190, *191*
Baked Onion Rings, 180, *181*
Balsamic-Braised Beet Greens, 168
Balsamic-Date Glaze, 8, 176, *177*
Bananas
    Banana-Chocolate Smoothie, 210, *211*
    Strawberry-Banana Nice Cream, *196*, 197
Beans, 122–123. *See also* Soybean foods
    Bean Patties with Harissa, 138, *139*
    Beans & Greens Quesadillas, *100*, 101
    benefits from, 138
    Black Bean Burgers, 88, *89*
    Black Bean Gazpacho Salad, 74, *75*
    Black Bean Sauce, *154*, 155
    Black Bean Soup with Quinoa & Kale, 56, *57*
    Black-Eyed Peas & Roasted Red Pepper Dip, 36, *37*
    cancer and, 138
    Chickpea & Vegetable Tagine, 124, *125*
    cooking tips for, 2

Curried Chickpea Wraps, 92, *93*
    Edamame Guacamole, 38, *39*
    Kale & White Bean Soup, 48, *49*
    Lemony Hummus, *32*, 33
    Lentil Bolognese, 150, *151*
    Lentil Shepherd's Pie, *132*, 133
    Louisiana Soy Curls, *136*, 137
    Moroccan Lentil Soup, 63
    Pesto Carrot Noodles with White Beans &
        Tomatoes, 106, *107*
    Quinoa Pilaf with Carrots & Chickpeas, *148*, 149
    shopping for, 229
    Skillet Sweet Potato Hash, *26*, 27
    Smoky Black-Eyed Peas & Collards, *126*, 127
    Spinach & Mushroom Black Bean Burritos, 94, *95*
    Summer Garden Gazpacho, 60, *61*
    Three-Bean Chili, 64, *65*
    Vegetable & Red Bean Gumbo, 54, *55*
    Yellow Rice & Black Beans with Broccoli, 152, *153*
    Yellow Split Pea Dal with Watercress, 134, *135*
Beets
    Beet Burgers, 98, *99*
    benefits from, 169
    for high blood pressure, 169
    Roasted Beets with Balsamic-Braised Beet Greens,
        168
Bell peppers. *See* Peppers
Beriberi, x
Berries
    Berry Chocolate Chia Pudding, 200, *201*
    Berry Drizzle, 16, *17*
    Blackberry Coulis, 192, *193*
    blueberries, xv
    Cherry-Berry Smoothie, *214*, 215
    Raspberry-Peach Crisp, *194*, 195
    Strawberry Balsamic Dressing, 84, *85*
    Strawberry-Banana Nice Cream, *196*, 197
    Two-Berry Pie with Pecan-Sunflower Crust, *202*,
        203
Beverages, 204–205. *See also* Smoothies
    Golden Chai, *208*, 209
    Lemon-Ginger Cooler, 206, *207*
    water, 206

Bisphenol A (BPA), 33
Black beans
    Black Bean Burgers, 88, *89*
    Black Bean Gazpacho Salad, 74, 75
    Black Bean Sauce, *154*, 155
    Black Bean Soup with Quinoa & Kale, 56, *57*
    Spinach & Mushroom Black Bean Burritos, 94, *95*
    Yellow Rice & Black Beans with Broccoli, 152, *153*
Black Women's Health Study, xviii
Blackberry Coulis, 192, *193*
Black-eyed peas
    Black-Eyed Peas & Roasted Red Pepper Dip, 36, *37*
    Smoky Black-Eyed Peas & Collards, *126*, 127
Blood cancers, xvii
Blood cells, xv
Blueberries, xv
Body mass index (BMI), xv
Bok choy, 128, *129*
BPA. *See* Bisphenol A
Brain diseases
    Alzheimer's disease, xiii–xiv
    high blood pressure and, xvi
    stroke, xiii–xiv, xvi
    whole-food, plant-based nutrition for, xiii–xiv
Braised Tempeh & Bok Choy with Spicy Ginger Sauce,
    128, *129*
Braising, 225
Breakfast, 10–11
    Burrito Breakfast Bake, 24, *25*
    Chocolate Oatmeal, *20*, 21
    French Toast with Berry Drizzle, 16, *17*
    Morning Grain Bowls, 22, *23*
    Skillet Sweet Potato Hash, *26*, 27
    Summertime Oatmeal, 12, *13*
    Superfood Breakfast Bites, *14*, 15
    Warm Pear Compote, 18, *19*
Breast cancer
    in African American women, xviii
    cholesterol and, xvii–xviii
    flaxseeds for, 15
    garlic for, 7
    soybean foods and, 98
    whole-food, plant-based nutrition for, xvii–xviii

Broccoli
>for cancer prevention, xvii
>for infections, preventing, xv
>lung diseases and, xiii
>Yellow Rice & Black Beans with Broccoli, 152, *153*

Broth, 6

Brown rice, x

Brownies, 198, *199*

Brussels sprouts, *166*, 167

Buckwheat Soba & Edamame with Almond Butter
>Sauce, 146

Buffalo Cauliflower, 7, 183

Burgers
>Beet Burgers, 98, *99*
>Black Bean Burgers, 88, *89*

Burritos
>Burrito Breakfast Bake, 24, *25*
>Spinach & Mushroom Black Bean Burritos, 94, *95*

C

Cabbage
>benefits from, 76
>Purple Cabbage Sauté, *172*, 173
>Sesame Purple Cabbage & Carrot Slaw, 76, 77

Campbell, Emeritus T. Colin, xii–xiii

Cancer
>blood, xvii
>breast, xvii–xviii, 7, 15, 98
>colon, xiv, 167
>digestive, xiv–xv, 7, 180
>EPIC study on, xv
>grilled or smoked meat and, xvii
>lung, xiii
>National Institutes of Health-AARP study on, xiv–
>>xv
>pancreatic cancer, xiv–xv, 7
>prostate cancer, xviii, 7
>rectal, xiv
>stomach, 7

Cancer-fighting foods
>beans as, 138

broccoli as, xvii
>Brussels sprouts as, 167
>cauliflower as, 115
>curry powder as, xiv
>flaxseeds as, 15
>garlic as, 7
>onions as, 180
>phytates, xiv
>soybean foods as, 98
>spinach as, 95
>turmeric as, xiv

Cardamom, 63

Carrageenan, 2

Carrots
>Lemon-Roasted Brussels Sprouts & Carrots with
>>Pecans, *166*, 167
>Pesto Carrot Noodles with White Beans &
>>Tomatoes, 106, *107*
>Quinoa Pilaf with Carrots & Chickpeas, *148*, 149
>Sesame Purple Cabbage & Carrot Slaw, 76, 77

Cashews, *104*, 105

Cauliflower
>Buffalo Cauliflower, 7, 183
>cancer and, 115
>Cauliflower Mash, *174*, 175
>Cauliflower Steaks with Chermoula Sauce, 118, *119*
>Chickpea & Cauliflower Curry, 130, *131*
>Curried Cauliflower Soup, *58*, 59
>Skillet Sweet Potato Hash, *26*, 27
>Whole Roasted Cauliflower with Lemon Tahini
>>Sauce, *114*, 115

Center for Alzheimer's Research, xiv

Ceylon cinnamon, 63

Chai, *208*, 209

Champion Vegetable Chili, 66, *67*

Cheesy Kale Crisps, 42, *43*

Chermoula Sauce, 118, *119*

Cherry-Berry Smoothie, *214*, 215

Chicken
>digestive cancers and, xv
>liver disease and, xvi
>toxic heavy metals in, xix

Chickpeas
    benefits from, 92
    Chickpea & Cauliflower Curry, 130, *131*
    Chickpea & Vegetable Tagine, 124, *125*
    Curried Chickpea Wraps, 92, *93*
    Lemony Hummus, *32*, 33
    Quinoa Pilaf with Carrots & Chickpeas, *148*, 149
    Smoky Roasted Chickpeas, 44, *45*
Chili
    Champion Vegetable Chili, 66, *67*
    Three-Bean Chili, 64, *65*
    variations of, 64
The China Study (Campbell), xii–xiii
China-Cornell-Oxford Project, xii–xiii
Chocolate
    Almond-Chocolate Truffles, *186*, 187
    Banana-Chocolate Smoothie, 210, *211*
    Berry Chocolate Chia Pudding, 200, *201*
    Chocolate Oatmeal, *20*, 21
    Fudgy No-Bake Brownies, 198, *199*
Cholesterol
    breast cancer and, xvii–xviii
    in coronary heart disease, xiii
    high, xiii
    kale and, 56
    kidney disease and, xvii
Chopped Vegetable Salad, *78*, 79
Chronic obstructive pulmonary disease (COPD), xiii
Cinnamon, 63
Cirrhosis, xvi
Collards
    Hoppin' John Stuffed Collard Rolls, 158, *159*
    Smoky Black-Eyed Peas & Collards, *126*, 127
Colon cancer, xiv, 167
Cookies, *188*, 189
Cooking methods, 225–226
Cooking tips, 2–3
COPD. *See* Chronic obstructive pulmonary disease
Coronary heart disease, x
    Campbell on, xii–xiii
    cholesterol in, xiii
    Esselstyn on, xiii
    Ornish on, xiii
    whole-food, plant-based nutrition for, xi, xii–xiii

Crohn's disease, 4
Culinary exploration, 30, 55
Culinary variety, 55
Curry powder
    as cancer-fighting food, xiv
    Chickpea & Cauliflower Curry, 130, *131*
    Curried Cauliflower Soup, *58*, 59
    Curried Chickpea Wraps, 92, *93*

D

Daily Dozen, xx–xxi. *See also specific recipes*
Dal, 134, *135*
Dates
    Bahri, 8
    Balsamic-Date Glaze, 8, 176, *177*
    date sugar, 3
    Date Syrup, 3, 5, 12, 16, 21, 22, *23*, 44, 70, 72, 76,
        80, 84, 190, 200, 209, 210, 215
    dried, 8
Depression, xviii
Desserts and sweets, 184–185
    Almond-Chocolate Truffles, *186*, 187
    Baked Apple Crumbles, 190, *191*
    Berry Chocolate Chia Pudding, 200, *201*
    Fresh Fruit Skewers with Blackberry Coulis, 192,
        193
    Fudgy No-Bake Brownies, 198, *199*
    No-Bake Oatmeal Walnut Cookies, *188*, 189
    Raspberry-Peach Crisp, *194*, 195
    Strawberry-Banana Nice Cream, *196*, 197
    Two-Berry Pie with Pecan-Sunflower Crust, *202*,
        203
Diabetes. *See* Type 2 diabetes
Diet
    disease and, viii–xi
    healthiest, x
    on holidays and special occasions, xi
Digestive cancers
    chicken and, xv
    onions and, 180
    stomach cancer, 7
    whole-food, plant-based nutrition for, xiv–xv

Dips and spreads
    Artichoke-Spinach Dip, 30, *31*
    Black-Eyed Peas & Roasted Red Pepper Dip, 36, *37*
    Edamame Guacamole, 38, *39*
    Lemony Hummus, *32*, 33
    Pumpkin Seed Dip, 35
    Summer Salsa, *40*, 41
Diseases. *See also specific diseases*
    diet and, viii–xi
    spinach for, 95
    turmeric for, 70
    whole-food, plant-based nutrition and, xi
    in womb, xiii
Doctors and medical care, viii–x, xix
Double-batch recipes, 2
Dressings. *See* Salads and dressings
Dried dates, 8
Dulse, 51

E

Edamame
    Buckwheat Soba & Edamame with Almond Butter
        Sauce, 146
    Edamame Guacamole, 38, *39*
Emphysema, xiii
EPIC study. *See* European Prospective Investigation into
        Cancer and Nutrition study
Esselstyn, Caldwell, Jr., xiii
European Prospective Investigation into Cancer and
        Nutrition (EPIC) study, xv

F

Fiber, xiv
Financial savings, ix
Flaxseeds
    for breast cancer, 15
    for high blood pressure, 15
    ways to use, 34
Food packaging, 33

Fortified refined grains, x
French toast
    French Toast with Berry Drizzle, 16, *17*
    Warm Pear Compote for, 18, *19*
Fresh Fruit Skewers with Blackberry Coulis, 192, *193*
Frozen foods, 227, 229
Fruit. *See also specific fruit*
    Fresh Fruit Skewers with Blackberry Coulis, 192,
        193
    shopping for, 229
    as snack, 41
Fudgy No-Bake Brownies, 198, *199*

G

Garbanzo beans. *See* Chickpeas
Garlic
    for cancer prevention, 7
    Garlic Caesar Dressing, *82*, 83
    Garlic Greens Sauté, 178
    Roasted Garlic, 6
Gazpacho
    Black Bean Gazpacho Salad, 74, *75*
    Summer Garden Gazpacho, 60, *61*
Ginger
    benefits from, 128
    Ginger Sesame Orange Dressing, 80, *81*
    Lemon-Ginger Cooler, 206, *207*
    Spicy Ginger Sauce, 128, *129*
Golden Chai, *208*, 209
Golden Gravy, 156–157, *157*
Golden Quinoa Tabouli, 70, *71*
Grains, 140–141
    Arugula Pesto Pasta with Roasted Vegetables, *160*,
        161
    Black Bean Soup with Quinoa & Kale, 56, *57*
    brown rice, x
    Buckwheat Soba & Edamame with Almond Butter
        Sauce, 146
    Chickpea & Vegetable Tagine, 124, *125*
    cooking tips for, 2
    fortified, x
    Golden Quinoa Tabouli, 70, *71*

Hoppin' John Stuffed Collard Rolls, 158, *159*

 Mac & Cheese, *142*, 143

 Morning Grain Bowls, 22, *23*

 Quinoa Pilaf with Carrots & Chickpeas, *148*, 149

 Red Quinoa Loaf with Golden Gravy, 156–157, *157*

 refined, x

 Roasted Vegetable Lasagna, *110*, 111

 shopping for, 229

 Stuffed Winter Squash with Black Bean Sauce, *154*, 155

 teff, 98

 Vegetable Unfried Rice, 144, *145*

 wheat, x

 white rice, x

 Whole Wheat Pasta with Lentil Bolognese, 150, *151*

 Yellow Rice & Black Beans with Broccoli, 152, *153*

Green Light foods, xi, 2

Greens. *See also specific greens*

 Balsamic-Braised Beet Greens, 168

 Beans & Greens Quesadillas, *100*, 101

 Garlic Greens Sauté, 178

 Portobellos & Greens on Toast, 121

 shopping for, 229

 Super Green Smoothie, 216, *217*

 ten ways to eat, 178

Guacamole, 38, *39*

Gumbo, 54, *55*

H

Harissa, 9, 138, *139*

Harvard University, xvii

Health

 Black Women's Health Study, xviii

 Iowa Women's Health Study, xvii

 power over, viii–ix

Healthiest diet, x

Healthy Hot Sauce, 8, 27, 52, 94, 127, 137, 158, 183

Heart disease. *See* Coronary heart disease

Heavy metals, xix

Hemp hearts, *82*, 83

Herbed Mushroom Gravy, 112, *113*

Hidradenitis suppurativa, 4

High blood pressure

 beets for, 169

 brain diseases and, xvi

 flaxseeds for, 15

 whole-food, plant-based nutrition for, xvi

High cholesterol, xiii

Holidays and special occasions, xi

Hoppin' John Stuffed Collard Rolls, 158, *159*

Hot sauce, 8

How Not to Die (Greger), viii–xi

 synopsis of, xii–xix

Hyperfiltration, of kidneys, xvii

Hypertension. *See* High blood pressure

I

Ice cream, *196*, 197

Ikeda, Kikunae, 5

Immune function, 121

Indian-Style Spinach and Tomatoes, 170, *171*

Infections, preventing, xv

Inflammation, xvii

Inflammatory conditions, 4, 70

Influenza, xv

Insulin, xv

Intraepithelial lymphocytes, xv

Iodine, 51

Iowa Women's Health Study, xvii

J

Jackfruit, *90*, 91

K

Kale

 benefits from, 56

 Black Bean Soup with Quinoa & Kale, 56, *57*

Cheesy Kale Crisps, 42, *43*

cholesterol and, 56

Ginger Sesame Orange Dressing, 80, *81*

Kale Salad with Avocado Goddess Dressing, 72, *73*

Kale & White Bean Soup, 48, *49*

Mango-Avocado-Kale Salad with Ginger Sesame Orange Dressing, 80, *81*

Kidney disease, xv, xvii

Kitchen techniques, 225–226

Kombu, 51

Lasagna, *110*, 111

Lead, xix

Legumes. *See* Beans

Lemons

    lemon juice, 3

    Lemon Tahini Sauce, *114*, 115

    Lemon-Ginger Cooler, 206, *207*

    Lemon-Roasted Brussels Sprouts & Carrots with Pecans, *166*, 167

    Lemony Hummus, *32*, 33

Lentils

    Lentil Bolognese, 150, *151*

    Lentil Shepherd's Pie, *132*, 133

    Moroccan Lentil Soup, 63

Lettuce, *96*, 97. *See also* Salads and Dressings

Leukemia, xvii

Lime juice, 3

Liver disease, xvi

Louisiana Soy Curls, *136*, 137

Lung cancer, xiii

Lung diseases, xiii

Lymphoma, xvii

M

Mac & Cheese, *142*, 143

Main dishes, 102–103

    Arugula Pesto Pasta with Roasted Vegetables, *160*, 161

    Bean Patties with Harissa, 138, *139*

    Braised Tempeh & Bok Choy with Spicy Ginger Sauce, 128, *129*

    Buckwheat Soba & Edamame with Almond Butter Sauce, 146

    Cauliflower Steaks with Chermoula Sauce, 118, *119*

    Chickpea & Cauliflower Curry, 130, *131*

    Chickpea & Vegetable Tagine, 124, *125*

    Hoppin' John Stuffed Collard Rolls, 158, *159*

    Lentil Shepherd's Pie, *132*, 133

    Louisiana Soy Curls, *136*, 137

    Mac & Cheese, *142*, 143

    Pesto Carrot Noodles with White Beans & Tomatoes, 106, *107*

    Portobellos & Greens on Toast, 121

    Quinoa Pilaf with Carrots & Chickpeas, *148*, 149

    Red Quinoa Loaf with Golden Gravy, 156–157, *157*

    Roasted Vegetable Lasagna, *110*, 111

    Smoky Black-Eyed Peas & Collards, *126*, 127

    Spaghetti Squash Arrabiata, 108, *109*

    Stuffed Portobellos with Herbed Mushroom Gravy, 112, *113*

    Stuffed Winter Squash with Black Bean Sauce, *154*, 155

    Vegetable Stacks with Tomato-Red Pepper Coulis, 116, *117*

    Vegetable Unfried Rice, 144, *145*

    Whole Roasted Cauliflower with Lemon Tahini Sauce, *114*, 115

    Whole Wheat Pasta with Lentil Bolognese, 150, *151*

    Yellow Rice & Black Beans with Broccoli, 152, *153*

    Yellow Split Pea Dal with Watercress, 134, *135*

    Zucchini Noodles with Avocado-Cashew Alfredo, *104*, 105

Mainstream medicine, viii–x, xii

Mango, 80, *81*

Medical radiation, xix

Medications, viii–x, xvi

Menstrual cramps, 128

Mercury, xix

Miso, 7

    Miso Soup with Spinach & Dulse, 51

Morning Grain Bowls, 22, *23*

Moroccan Lentil Soup, 63

Multiple myeloma, xvii

Mushrooms

    benefits from, 113, 121

Portobellos & Greens on Toast, 121
Spinach & Mushroom Black Bean Burritos, 94, *95*
Stuffed Portobellos with Herbed Mushroom Gravy, 112, *113*

N

NAFLD. *See* Nonalcoholic fatty liver disease
National Institutes of Health-AARP study, xiv–xv
Natural killer cells, xv
No-Bake Oatmeal Walnut Cookies, *188*, 189
Nonalcoholic fatty liver disease (NAFLD), xvi
Nutrition. *See* Diet; Whole-food, plant-based nutrition
Nutritional yeast, 4, 44
NutritionFacts.org, viii, xii
Nuts and seeds
    almond butter, 2
    Almond Butter Sauce, 146
    Almond Milk, xi, 2
    Almond-Chocolate Truffles, *186*, 187
    benefits from, 108, 146
    cashews, *104*, 105
    cooking, 108
    flaxseeds, 15, 34
    Nutty Parm, 4, 105, 106, 108, 111, 150, 161
    pecans, *166*, 167, *202*, 203
    Pistachio-Spinach Salad with Strawberry Balsamic Dressing, 84, *85*
    Pumpkin Seed Dip, 35
    raw, 108
    Sesame Purple Cabbage & Carrot Slaw, 76, 77
    shopping for, 229
    soaking and blending, 225
    Three-Seed Crackers, 34
    walnuts, 106, *188*, 189

O

Oatmeal, xi
    Chocolate Oatmeal, *20*, 21
    No-Bake Oatmeal Walnut Cookies, *188*, 189
    Summertime Oatmeal, 12, *13*
    Warm Pear Compote for, 18, *19*
Oats, x
Okra, 54, *55*
Onions, 180, *181*
Oranges, 80, *81*
Ornish, Dean, x, xiii, xviii

P

Pancreatic cancer, xiv–xv, 7
Pantry, 227–229
Paprika, 63
Parchment paper, 225
Parkinson's disease
    peppers for, 117
    whole-food, plant-based nutrition for, xix
Pasta
    Arugula Pesto Pasta with Roasted Vegetables, *160*, 161
    Buckwheat Soba & Edamame with Almond Butter Sauce, 146
    Mac & Cheese, *142*, 143
    Roasted Vegetable Lasagna, *110*, 111
    shopping for, 229
    Whole Wheat Pasta with Lentil Bolognese, 150, *151*
Pawpaw, 80
PCB. *See* Polychlorinated biphenyl
Peaches, *194*, 195
Pears, 18, *19*
Peas, 176
Pecans
    Lemon-Roasted Brussels Sprouts & Carrots with Pecans, *166*, 167
    Two-Berry Pie with Pecan-Sunflower Crust, *202*, 203
Peppers
    benefits from, 117
    Black-Eyed Peas & Roasted Red Pepper Dip, 36, *37*
    Harissa, 9
    Healthy Hot Sauce, 8
    for Parkinson's disease, 117
    roasting, 9

Summer Salsa, *40*, 41

Tomato-Red Pepper Coulis, 116, *117*

Yellow Pepper Béarnaise, 164, *165*

Permanente, Kaiser, xi

Pesto

Arugula Pesto Pasta with Roasted Vegetables, *160*, 161

Pesto Carrot Noodles with White Beans & Tomatoes, 106, *107*

Phytates, xiv

Pie

Pumpkin Pie Smoothie, 212, *213*

Two-Berry Pie with Pecan-Sunflower Crust, *202*, 203

Pistachio-Spinach Salad with Strawberry Balsamic Dressing, 84, *85*

Plant pigments, 56, 59, 227

The Plant-Based Diet: A Healthier Way to Eat (Permanente), xi

Pneumonia, xv

Polychlorinated biphenyl (PCB), xix

Polyps, 70

Popcorn, 44

Portobellos & Greens on Toast, 121

Potassium, xiv

Pregnancy, xiii

Prepping tips, 2

Pritikin, Nathan, xi, xii

Processed foods, x, xi

Prostate cancer, xviii, 7

Pudding, 200, *201*

Pumpkin Pie Smoothie, 212, *213*

Pumpkin Seed Dip, 35

Purple Cabbage Sauté, *172*, 173

Q

Quesadillas, *100*, 101

Quinoa

Black Bean Soup with Quinoa & Kale, 56, *57*

Chickpea & Vegetable Tagine, 124, *125*

Golden Quinoa Tabouli, 70, *71*

Quinoa Pilaf with Carrots & Chickpeas, *148*, 149

Red Quinoa Loaf with Golden Gravy, 156–157, *157*

R

Ranch Dressing, 7, 183

Raspberry-Peach Crisp, *194*, 195

Raw nuts and seeds, 108

Rectal cancer, xiv

Red beans, 54, *55*

Red Light foods, xi, 2

Red Quinoa Loaf with Golden Gravy, 156–157, *157*

Refined grains, x

Rice

brown, x

Vegetable Unfried Rice, 144, *145*

white, x

Yellow Rice & Black Beans with Broccoli, 152, *153*

Roasted Asparagus with Yellow Pepper Béarnaise, 164, *165*

Roasted Beets with Balsamic-Braised Beet Greens, 168

Roasted Garlic, 6, 7, 35

Roasted Vegetable Lasagna, *110*, 111

Roasting, 9, 225

S

Saffron, xviii

Salads and dressings, 68–69

Black Bean Gazpacho Salad, 74, *75*

Chopped Vegetable Salad, 78, *79*

Golden Quinoa Tabouli, 70, *71*

Kale Salad with Avocado Goddess Dressing, 72, *73*

Mango-Avocado-Kale Salad with Ginger Sesame Orange Dressing, 80, *81*

Pistachio-Spinach Salad with Strawberry Balsamic Dressing, 84, *85*

Ranch Dressing, 7, 79, 183

salad bar, 78

Sesame Purple Cabbage & Carrot Slaw, 76, *77*

Super Salad with Garlic Caesar Dressing & Hemp Hearts, *82*, 83

Salsa, *40*, 41

Salt, 7

Sample menus, 220–223

Sandwiches, burgers, and wraps, 86–87

    Beans & Greens Quesadillas, *100*, 101

    Beet Burgers, 98, *99*

    Black Bean Burgers, 88, *89*

    Curried Chickpea Wraps, 92, *93*

    Sloppy Jacks, *90*, 91

    Spinach & Mushroom Black Bean Burritos, 94, *95*

    Veracruz Tempeh Lettuce Wraps, *96*, 97

Sauces

    Almond Butter Sauce, 146

    Arrabiata, 108, *109*

    Avocado-Cashew Alfredo, *104*, 105

    Balsamic-Date Glaze, 8, *176*, 177

    Berry Drizzle, 16, *17*

    Black Bean Sauce, *154*, 155

    Blackberry Coulis, 192, *193*

    Chermoula Sauce, 118, *119*

    Golden Gravy, 156–157, *157*

    Harissa, 9, 138, *139*

    Herbed Mushroom Gravy, 112, *113*

    Lemon Tahini Sauce, *114*, 115

    Lentil Bolognese, 150, *151*

    Spicy Ginger Sauce, 128, *129*

    Tomato-Red Pepper Coulis, 116, *117*

    Umami Sauce, xxii, 5, 27

    Warm Pear Compote, 18, *19*

    Yellow Pepper Béarnaise, 164, *165*

Savory Spice Blend, xxii, 4, 6, 7, 9, 24, 27, 30, 35, 36, 38, 41, 44, 48, 51, 52, 54, 56, 59, 60, 63, 64, 66, 70, 72, 83, 88, 91, 92, 94, 101, 108, 115, 127, 137, 143, 149, 167, 180, 183

Seaweed, 51

Seeds. *See* Nuts and seeds

Sesame Purple Cabbage & Carrot Slaw, 76, 77

Shopping, 227–229

Side dishes, 162–163

    Baked Onion Rings, 180, *181*

    Buffalo Cauliflower, 7, 183

    Cauliflower Mash, *174*, 175

    Garlic Greens Sauté, 178

    Indian-Style Spinach and Tomatoes, 170, *171*

    Lemon-Roasted Brussels Sprouts & Carrots with Pecans, *166*, 167

    Purple Cabbage Sauté, *172*, 173

    Roasted Asparagus with Yellow Pepper Béarnaise, 164, *165*

    Roasted Beets with Balsamic-Braised Beet Greens, 168

    Stuffed Sweet Potatoes, 8, 176, *177*

Silicone mats, 225

Simmering, 225

60 Minutes, xi

Skillet Sweet Potato Hash, *26*, 27

Sloppy Jacks, *90*, 91

Smoked meat, xvii

Smoked paprika, 63

Smoky Roasted Chickpeas, 44, *45*

Smoothies

    Banana-Chocolate Smoothie, 210, *211*

    Cherry-Berry Smoothie, *214*, 215

    Pumpkin Pie Smoothie, 212, *213*

    Super Green Smoothie, 216, *217*

    V-12 Vegetable Blast, *218*, 219

Snacks, 28–29

    Artichoke-Spinach Dip, 30, *31*

    Black-Eyed Peas & Roasted Red Pepper Dip, 36, *37*

    Cheesy Kale Crisps, 42, *43*

    Edamame Guacamole, 38, *39*

    fruit, as, 41

    Lemony Hummus, *32*, 33

    popcorn, 44

    Pumpkin Seed Dip, 35

    Smoky Roasted Chickpeas, 44, *45*

    Summer Salsa, *40*, 41

    Three-Seed Crackers, 34

Soda, xvi

Sodium, 7

Soups and chilies, 46–47

    Black Bean Soup with Quinoa & Kale, 56, *57*

    Champion Vegetable Chili, 66, *67*

    Curried Cauliflower Soup, *58*, 59

    Kale & White Bean Soup, 48, *49*

    Miso Soup with Spinach & Dulse, 51

    Moroccan Lentil Soup, 63

    Spicy Asian Vegetable Soup, 52, *53*

Summer Garden Gazpacho, 60, *61*

Three-Bean Chili, 64, *65*

Vegetable Broth, 6

Vegetable & Red Bean Gumbo, 54, *55*

Soybean foods, 98

    Braised Tempeh & Bok Choy with Spicy Ginger Sauce, 128, *129*

    Buckwheat Soba & Edamame with Almond Butter Sauce, 146

    Edamame Guacamole, 38, *39*

    Louisiana Soy Curls, *136*, 137

    miso, 7, 51

    steaming tempeh, 225

    Veracruz Tempeh Lettuce Wraps, *96*, 97

Spaghetti Squash Arrabiata, 108, *109*

Spices. *See also* Curry powder; Turmeric

    cardamom, 63

    cinnamon, 63

    cooking tips for, 2

    cooking with, 63

    paprika, 63

    saffron, xviii

    Savory Spice Blend, xxii, 4, 27

Spicy Asian Vegetable Soup, 52, *53*

Spicy Ginger Sauce, 128, *129*

Spinach

    Artichoke-Spinach Dip, 30, *31*

    as cancer-fighting food, 95

    for diseases, 95

    Indian-Style Spinach and Tomatoes, 170, *171*

    Miso Soup with Spinach & Dulse, 51

    Pistachio-Spinach Salad with Strawberry Balsamic Dressing, 84, *85*

    Spinach & Mushroom Black Bean Burritos, 94, *95*

    using, 94

Spreads. *See* Dips and spreads

Squash

    Pumpkin Pie Smoothie, 212, *213*

    Spaghetti Squash Arrabiata, 108, *109*

    Stuffed Winter Squash with Black Bean Sauce, *154*, 155

    Zucchini Noodles with Avocado-Cashew Alfredo, *104*, 105

Steaming, 225

Stir-frying, 226

Stomach cancer, 7

Storage containers, 33

Strawberries

    Strawberry Balsamic Dressing, 84, *85*

    Strawberry-Banana Nice Cream, *196*, 197

Stroke, xiii–xiv, xvi

Stuffed Portobellos with Herbed Mushroom Gravy, 112, *113*

Stuffed Sweet Potatoes, 8, 176, *177*

Sugar, date, 3

Suicidal depression, xviii

Summer Garden Gazpacho, 60, *61*

Summer Salsa, *40*, 41

Summertime Oatmeal, 12, *13*

Super Green Smoothie, 216, *217*

Super Salad with Garlic Caesar Dressing & Hemp Hearts, *82*, 83

Superfood Breakfast Bites, *14*, 15

Sweet Potatoes

    Burrito Breakfast Bake, 24, *25*

    Skillet Sweet Potato Hash, *26*, 27

    Stuffed Sweet Potatoes, 8, 176, *177*

Sweets. *See* Desserts and sweets

Syrup, 3, 22, *23*

T

Tabouli, 70, *71*

Tagine, 124, *125*

Tahini, *114*, 115

Teff, 98

Tempeh

    Braised Tempeh & Bok Choy with Spicy Ginger Sauce, 128, *129*

    steaming, 225

    Veracruz Tempeh Lettuce Wraps, *96*, 97

Tetra Pak, 24

Three-Bean Chili, 64, *65*

Three-Seed Crackers, 34

Time-saving cooking tips, 2

Tomato products, 229

Tomatoes

    Indian-Style Spinach and Tomatoes, 170, *171*

Pesto Carrot Noodles with White Beans &
    Tomatoes, 106, *107*
Summer Garden Gazpacho, 60, *61*
Summer Salsa, *40*, 41
Tomato-Red Pepper Coulis, 116, *117*
Tortillas, 229
Toxic heavy metals, xix
Traffic-light classification system, x–xi, 2
Triglyceride levels, 8
Turmeric
    as cancer-fighting food, xiv
    for diseases, 70
    in French Toast with Berry Drizzle, 16
    in Golden Gravy, 156–157, *157*
    in Golden Quinoa Tabouli, 70, *71*
    ten ways to eat, 70
Two-Berry Pie with Pecan-Sunflower Crust, *202*, 203
Type 2 diabetes
    diet and, viii–ix
    insulin in, xv
    kidney disease and, xv
    medications for, viii–x, xvi
    type 2, viii–ix
    whole-food, plant-based nutrition for, xv–xvi

U

Umami, 5
Umami Sauce, xxii, 5, 27, 64, 121, 128, 133, 144, 146,
    155, 173,

V

V-12 Vegetable Blast, *218*, 219
Veganism, x
Vegetable Broth, 5, 6, 30, 48, 51, 52, 54, 56, 59, 63, 64,
    66, 105, 106, 112, 124, 128, 130, 133, 134,
    137, 143, 152, 155, 157, 164, 173, 178, 226
Vegetable & Red Bean Gumbo, 54, *55*
Vegetable Stacks with Tomato-Red Pepper Coulis, 116,
    117
Vegetable Unfried Rice, 144, *145*
Vegetarianism, x
Veracruz Tempeh Lettuce Wraps, *96*, 97
Vinegar, 5, 73
    Balsamic-Braised Beet Greens, 168
    Balsamic-Date Glaze, 8, 176, *177*
    Strawberry Balsamic Dressing, 84, *85*
Vision loss, xv

W

Walnuts, 106
    No-Bake Oatmeal Walnut Cookies, *188*, 189
Warm Pear Compote, 18, *19*
Water, 206
Watercress, 134, *135*
Water-sauté, 226
Weight, xv, 92
Wheat. *See* Grains
White beans
    Kale & White Bean Soup, 48, *49*
    Pesto Carrot Noodles with White Beans &
        Tomatoes, 106, *107*
White blood cells, xv
White rice, x
Whole Roasted Cauliflower with Lemon Tahini Sauce,
    114, 115
Whole-food, plant-based nutrition, x–xi
    for blood cancers, xvii
    for brain diseases, xiii–xiv
    for breast cancer, xvii–xviii
    for coronary heart disease, xi, xii–xiii
    for digestive cancers, xiv–xv
    diseases and, xi
    for high blood pressure, xvi
    for infections, xv
    for kidney disease, xvii
    for liver disease, xvi
    for lung diseases, xiii
    for Parkinson's disease, xix
    for prostate cancer, xviii

for suicidal depression, xviii

for type 2 diabetes, xv–xvi

weight and, xv

Womb, xiii

Wraps

Beans & Greens Quesadillas, *100*, 101

Curried Chickpea Wraps, 92, *93*

Spinach & Mushroom Black Bean Burritos, 94, *95*

Veracruz Tempeh Lettuce Wraps, *96*, 97

Y

Yeast, nutritional, 4, 44

Yellow Light foods, xi, 2

Yellow Pepper Béarnaise, 164, *165*

Yellow Rice & Black Beans with Broccoli, 152, *153*

Z

Zucchini, *104*, 105

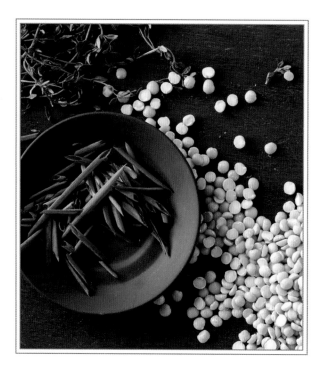